"From my experience as a physician, nothing is more devastating for the patient and family than to learn that medical teams do not always agree on the best course of action -- especially tough when the disease is life-threatening."
— TERRY B STROM, MD, Professor of Medicine at Harvard Medical School and Co-Director of The Transplant Institute @ Beth Israel Deaconess Medical Center

***

"The story of a father's courage, a daughter's strength and a very personal triumph for medical research."
— P. MICHAEL CONN, Ph.D, Oregon Health & Science University and co-author of *The Animal Research War*

***

"Paul McLean bravely takes us into every parent's nightmare—a healthy child, a mysterious disease, a young life suddenly at risk—and shows us how to come through it. Blood Lines will give comfort and answers to anyone who finds themselves in need of hope in the midst of chaos and tragedy. This is a book of miracles: about how a family, community, and medicine collaborated on curing a child -- told by a father who lived it."
— SUSAN SENATOR, author of *Making Peace With Autism, The Autism Mom's Survival Guide*

***

"When a parent's worst nightmare occurs, the desperate illness and possible death of their child, most of us have no words to describe it. As a writer Paul McLean tells his journey with honesty, an open heart, and his idiosyncratic humor. This is not a book to be read in public or just before going to bed. I wept, I laughed, I nodded in recognition, and I wept some more."
— REV. DR. JIM SHERBLOM, First Parish in Brookline, Massachusetts

BLOOD LINES

Fatherhood, faith and
love in the time of stem cells

By Paul C. McLean

PUBLISHER'S INFORMATION

EBookBakery Books

Author contact: paul@paulcmclean.com
Blogs by Paul McLean:
medicalethicsandme.org
paulcmclean.com

ISBN 978-1-938517-23-5

Cover design: Kristin Leader
www.kleaderdesign.com

ACKNOWLEDGMENTS

While researching "Blood Lines," I described to my wife some of the scientists and others I discovered in Douglas Starr's "Blood" and Stephen S. Hall's "A Commotion in the Blood." And she said, "It seems like you're wanting to know who to thank." In many ways this book itself is an acknowledgment, an accounting of gratitude I'll never express sufficiently, or to all who deserve it.

In writing this book, though, authors Starr and Hall were invaluable in my understanding of the 20th century science that made a cure possible. Physician-authors Jerome Groopman and Siddhartha Mukherjee were extraordinary sources for appreciating clinical and research science in all its ambiguous glory.

For reading drafts and for their advice, encouragement and creative feedback: Gerry Leader, Lucy Aptekar, Susan Senator, Adam Strom, Sandy Smith Garcez, Dr. Terry B. Strom and Brent McLean. For literary insight and guidance: Deanne Urmy. For editing with the eyes of an eagle and heart of a patient advocate: Michela Moscufo. For editing, publishing and marketing guidance: Lisa Tener. For being a godsend to a self-publishing writer: Michael Grossman. And for her support, feedback and a cover that so artfully tells my story: Kristin Leader.

Of course, Jody and J lived this story with me. I could not have written it without their love and support.

Dedication

To Jody and J.
All the way to Fife.

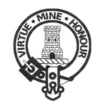

Foreword

"Blood Lines" written by Paul McLean should be required reading for medical care givers as well as for parents whose child is diagnosed with a life-threatening, albeit potentially curable, illness.

The McLean family is of course shaken when they learn that their 7-year-old daughter has developed aplastic anemia. In this somewhat unusual condition, bone marrow function is defective. As the ability of the bone marrow to produce red and white blood cells as well as platelets is seriously compromised, their daughter becomes increasingly anemic and prone to infection and bleeding.

Bolstered by spiritual and intellectual resources and living very close to the Harvard Medical School complex, treatment is initiated and accompanied by considerable camaraderie between the family and the medical team providing care. The family comes together to provide loving and, over time, 24/7 care for their daughter. Moreover, the care rendered by health care providers is tender and thoughtful.

Unfortunately the standard treatment for aplastic anemia fails to produce significant benefit and attention turns to bone marrow, or blood stem cell transplantation, as the next step. This offers the promise of cure but also carries considerable risk over a prolonged period of treatment, hospitalization and recovery.

This unwanted and unexpected news created tremendous angst but also determination by the parents to help their remarkably resilient daughter get through this difficult emotional and medical hurdle. The emotional impact upon the parents is profound.

Successful treatment requires identification of a "good" match for certain genetic traits between the donor and recipient and upon the imposition of treatments that prevent recipient immune cells from rejecting the donor transplant; donor immune cells migrating from the transplant from attacking recipient tissue (graft versus host disease); and toxicity from the rather harsh measures used to block this two-way immunologic warfare.

From my experience as a physician, nothing is more devastating for the patient and family than to learn that medical teams do not always agree on the best course of action—especially tough when the disease is life-threatening. Regretfully this type of soul-shattering news is what the family heard. The transplant teams in Boston and Seattle, both highly regarded, did not agree upon the details of treatment for patients receiving a stem cell transplant and this breech was particularly wide in treatment of patients with aplastic anemia.

Treatment for stem cell transplantation was undergoing clinical testing, new treatments were being introduced into clinical trials, and there was widespread reconsideration of treatment strategies. Unfortunately the clinical trials had not been completed and there was considerable doubt as to the best course of action.

At the time, clinical testing of low and higher intensity radiation treatments, to prevent GVHD, were ongoing but definitive answers were not in hand. The superb transplant program in Seattle, pioneers in stem cell transplantation, championed low-intensity radiation while the Harvard program was not yet convinced of the merit of this approach until clinical testing produced a definitive answer.

The family was convinced, correctly as later events prove, that low-intensity radiation was the way to go. The conflict arising between the family and their physicians at the famed medical center, located in walking distance of their home, caused incalculable pain and no small measure of anger. Part of the problem was the manner in which the principal caregiver at Harvard delivered the news and resolve not to consider another path.

The main issue, however, was a clash in judgment as to whether another institution's new and highly promising approach, albeit not entirely proven, should be applied absent certainty of benefit and without a randomized trial to measure the value of the new treatment against the current standard. With great sacrifice the family went to seek care in Seattle and the story has a very happy ending.

This painful and highly personal story gives insight into the forces that can place patient and physician in conflict and suggests means to minimize the pain and maintain a productive relationship even if the patient care must be transferred to other doctors and institutions.

Terry B. Strom, MD, Harvard Medical School

AUTHOR'S NOTE

Dr. Terry Strom has devoted a professional lifetime to the science of immune tolerance, to understanding the meticulous negotiation that is pivotal to successful transplant, whether of a live organ or stem cells.

He has argued before Congress to get funding for cyclosporine, the immune-suppressant drug which transformed transplant by chemically enforcing a peace between host and the new cells or organ. That is, it transformed the fatal into the treatable and gave new life to humans facing a death sentence.

At its best, transplantation trades the cloud of a terminal or life-threatening problem for a new and unpredictable reality and additional days on the planet.

Devotion to tolerance of a different kind has been the life's work of Margot Strom, Terry's wife and founder of the educational nonprofit Facing History and Ourselves.

To have the Strom name connected with my story is a profound gift. That his own life has now been extended by transplantation of his own stem cells—well, the karmic justice gives this author chills.

The people and events of this book are real. Select names have been changed or omitted out of respect.

Blood Lines, as any respectable dictionary will tell you, is one word. The layers of meaning demanded more space, though, so I went with two. My inner copy editor calls this a typo, intentional though it might be. But if the events of this story taught me nothing else, they taught me a tolerance for ambiguity.

Chapter One

How to Stop a Nosebleed

We sat on the grass, tilted our heads back and waited for the fireworks. Staring expectantly into the darkening sky over a distant Edinburgh Castle, my wife and I anticipated something extraordinary to explode the day back to life. This would be worth it, we assured our daughter, who didn't share our enthusiasm. She wasn't assured, but then, she'd been contrarian of late. *Wonder where she got that?*

Fireworks shows, the good ones, combine the expected with the unexpected. A fading speck seems to expire and disappear, then illuminates earth and sky with a percussive blast. But how spectacular could a Scottish display be, even one punctuating the close of the Edinburgh Festival? Those things cost money, you know, and the Scots are thrifty folk, as my father would say, in jest or awareness or self-deprecating hybrid. A clan descendant, he was. Cheap is in my very marrow.

The fireworks backlit the castle, creating moments at once ancient and immediate. *This is where we're from,* I told J.

In July 1998, Jody and I lay in our bed in our hilltop condominium in Brookline, Massachusetts, and introduced our infant daughter to her first fireworks show. J mostly slept, but we listened to a live broadcast of the Boston Pops, and could see and hear the explosions over the Charles River from our bedroom window. J, nearly seven months old, snuggled between us in a moment that could be no more seared into my memory if I'd held a lit fuse in my palm a second too long. The distant explosions lit J's angelic face and beautifully bald head as she breathed steadily and peacefully, oblivious to the blasts. Far removed from the riverside crowds, we had our own show, a private celebration of this young life, so full of promise, sleeping peacefully between us.

Seven years later, she'd grown up so much, as we sat in an Edinburgh park, at slight elevation, waiting for the events to unfold before us, staring off toward what J once described with a toddler's wonderment as *the horizon in the distance.*

I told her about buying sparklers as a kid. I'd light them, get a cheap thrill and wreak no pyrotechnic havoc whatsoever. They were the only ones my parents let me handle. Advertised as safe and sane, they were boring. Same with Snakes. You'd light the little black pellet and watch it sizzle and make like an ashen Slinky. A conservative kid, from conservative blood, I liked the more showy displays, but didn't want my fingerprints on them, or my actual fingers detonating along with them. Let someone who knew what they were doing handle those, someone more carefree than I.

Friends were inclined toward the riskier kind, and I'd get my kicks vicariously through them, like that Roman candle that flew upward maybe 20 feet, then made a hard right into the neighbor's shake shingle. We got the hose and extinguished it without event. Or that M-80 that lit up the intersection in our residential L.A. suburb. We sprinted away and felt the impact of the blast, saw night turn to day behind us, then hid behind cars and bushes during the obligatory patrol by the town police. It was exciting, but I wondered why we were doing something you could get in trouble for. I sought deniability that held up in the confessional.

We didn't go out of our way to find fireworks in Edinburgh. It was merely good timing that our vacation was ending as the Edinburgh Festival drew to a close. Jody participated in a psychological conference in Edinburgh, ostensibly our reason for going, though I'd dreamt of traveling to Scotland for years, a dream that once included taking Dad to Saint Andrews and walking the Old Course, father and son, like golf legends Old Tom and Young Tom Morris.

Old Tom outlived his son, a sad fate. Many times we sat under a vintage photograph of them at Dad's favorite coffee shop, known for its early bird specials. Then Dad died, and took the Scotland dream with him. A few days before the Edinburgh fireworks, as I played the Old Course with three Germans nice enough to let me crash their tee time, Dad was very much present. I could almost smell the smoke from his pipe tobacco, see him smile proudly at the 20-footer with a big left-to-right break that

I rolled for birdie on No. 7, sense his disappointment and mild admonishment when I swore at a muffed 8-iron on the Road Hole. If I'd putted like him, I'd have broken 80. R.J. McLean wouldn't have three-jabbed one of those greens. Not one.

I also felt him at Duart Castle, the ancestral Maclean home on the Isle of Mull in Western Scotland. The stairs would have been hell on his knees, but he would have taken his time and loved the climb anyway. My daughter and I signed the official Maclean Clan guestbook at Duart Castle. *Our castle*, we called it. The chief of the clan lives there part of the year. Sean Connery, said to be a Maclean somewhere along the line, filmed scenes from the movie *Entrapment* at Duart Castle. Jody and I rented the video. Pardon my Gaelic, but the movie sucked, other than its views of the castle.

The Isle of Mull is accessible by ferry from the port of Oban, where we stayed in an inn run by a McLean with floors covered in the clan's tartan. Breakfast was in a room crammed with tchotchkes, clearly a genetic trait, and a piano inexplicably featuring the sheet music to "Highway to Hell."

Oban is known for its single malt, a highway I've been known to travel, and Jody and I managed a tour of the distillery, but the castle was our destination. We drove our rental van onto the ferry, to better explore the island and fit in a side trip to Lochbuie, with a bay of stunning beauty and ruins of another ancient Maclean homestead. Or McLean homestead. Same thing. Over many centuries, the Clan MacGhille-Eoin, Gaelic for son of the servant of John, survived without a copy editor.

Walking the alternately rocky and verdant grounds of Duart Castle, J and I kept finding dark, furry caterpillars and joked that they were R.J.'s eyebrows. J, being her mother's daughter, tired of the joke. When I saw more of the hairy critters while playing 36 holes in Nairn, the last nine with three local seniors whose thick brogues only my father would've understood, I smiled and said nothing.

Duart Castle is on a promontory on the eastern tip of Mull. In 1653, Cromwell's forces watched from the rocky shore as 22 friends died aboard the wrecked Swan. Or Swann. (Vowels and consonants dropping in and out without rhyme or reason may not be exclusively a Maclean thing.)

7

Cromwell's fleet anchored off the point and set about to claiming the castle and all inside, which amounted to none at all, as the McLeans had anticipated trouble and gotten out. The ability to see trouble on the horizon was not passed down to me, as I soon would learn. The Cromwell forces, anchored and protected from the prevailing southwesterly winds, were surprised by a northwesterly gale that sank three of the six in the fleet. Two held cargo; the Swan held fighters.

The castle was musty in places, not that I thought about it then. Back in that lifetime, before my daughter's blood line turned on her, mold and mildew were a shower-curtain embarrassment. Blood was a figurative thing, a line I could trace by flying to Scotland or Ireland, or even to Canada, or just by reading Dad's hand-written account. Blood was a metaphor for poets and songwriters. A platelet was a piece of armor with a Clan Maclean insignia on it: Virtue Mine Honor.

Of course the castle was musty; the place was old and perched by the sea. But I wasn't thinking in those terms.

I wouldn't have it back, but I miss that naivete: the feeling that this world is a safe place to raise my child, to introduce another generation of McLean. But that's not my world anymore. The world I inherited—in which everyone is the enemy, the carrier, the potential source of infection and threat to life—demands reverence and gratitude for the singular pulse of the moment, and denies assumption of anything beyond it. I suspect that world is the one I've always lived in, however blissfully unaware. *Be here now*, Ram Dass said. I'd heard it before; I get it now.

Duart Castle was a ruin for centuries, but in the early 1900s the clan undertook an impressive restoration. *That must've cost a bit,* as Dad would have said. They opened the castle for tourists, and hold the occasional clan reunion. The ticket seller tells visitors, no matter the surname, not to bother the chief. I'd like to knock on the door, introduce myself, a highlander raised under a palm tree, and suggest the clan invest in dehumidifiers.

But we didn't bother the chief. We hiked out to the rocks near where the Swan went down. We poked our heads in dungeons. J and I signed the book, our signatures following assorted Macleans, McLains, Lanes, McGranes, McClains and other variations, each one a cousin in one way or another. There were two books, but only McLeans signed the clan book. My wife signed the just-visiting, I'm-with-them book. You don't take the name, you pay the price. Or the piper, as the case may be.

Closing my eyes now, I can see fireworks lighting up Duart Castle, illuminating a history I'd only just tasted and lending color to my daughter's pale cheeks. But those ones aren't real. The real fireworks were over Edinburgh Castle, and on a late-summer night in 2005, as my wife and daughter and I watched from a crowded park, the fireworks seemed a fitting conclusion and celebration of our vacation in Scotland, where my paternal grandmother was born a Mooney, from where my great great great great grandfather John McLean Sr. and his son John Jr. sailed in 1790, and where my father always wanted to visit but never got around to it. Surely on that September night in Edinburgh, with the heavens illuminated and percussive, and the pipers and my fellow knights of the single malt out in force, the demons were already at work inside my daughter.

How long they'd been at work, no one can truly say. But within days, back home in Brookline, Massachusetts, those little dark bumps my wife and I treated as something of a curiosity of no particular concern gave way to large, inexplicable bruises as J's complexion turned a ghostly pale. Before long her first CBC would reveal just how depleted her blood supply had become. Before long that bloody nose, which stopped suddenly on a bus ride back from the Edinburgh Zoo, would return and show no signs of ceasing until an emergency room doctor at Boston Children's Hospital cauterized her nostril with a couple of long matchsticks that looked like Fourth of July sparklers. I'm sure there's a different name for them, but they looked like sparklers, and burned like sparklers. Oh, how they burned. My seven-year-old daughter's face told me just how much they burned.

I can't summon up the memory of my daughter's cries that night in the ER; I must've put them away in some dank and distant space, some musty dungeon in the bowels of an ancient castle. I can see my wife holding her, comforting her. J must have been calling out for me to make them stop what they were doing. I'm sure she called out something like that, because I remember thinking I would make them stop if only I could. If only I had the ability. But that was the night when my parenting skills, the limits of my protective abilities, were laid bare. I felt useless, a feeling I would become painfully familiar with, though I never got used to it. A simple fact: I couldn't stop the bleeding. Jody rocked J, and I slipped out of the ER room and cried.

Did you really cry? J asked me later when she wanted to hear my version of the story of the beginning of her illness. I told her I really did. *Why?* she wanted to know. *Because I wished it could be me on that table instead of you. Because I was scared,* I said. *How scared?* she asked. *Scared as I've ever been,* I said.

Days earlier in Edinburgh, as the fireworks gave the contemporary horizon its medieval silhouette, I didn't know what a neutrophil was, let alone that I needed thousands of them to fight off a run-of-the-mill infection or that my daughter's supply was fast depleting. That a T cell, a killer T cell, could become so deranged and traitorous as to attack its own host. That a platelet, unlike a father, could stop the bleeding, if there were enough of them. CBC was an acronym for a TV network in the country where my siblings were born; now it's a complete blood count. GVH sounded like a PBS station in Boston with a habit of interrupting Roy Orbison in black and white with pleas for money; now it's what happens to just about everyone who gets a bone marrow transplant, the survivors and the others alike.

Acronyms have changed. Everything has changed. It's all about blood now. Fireworks are stem cells exploding into blood products—red cells to move protein and oxygen around the body, white cells to chase down infections, platelets to stick their finger in the leaky hole. Give me safe and sane. Now. Please.

J complained that last night in Edinburgh of being tired, but she tended to do that when her parents wanted her to join them in an activity she'd rather skip to stay home and watch TV, like that long hike up a misty mountain in the highlands near Torridon. Jody remembers J had a bloody nose that night, too. J complained that the midges were bothering her. In Scotland, she became obsessed with midges, tiny biting bugs that would be mythical were they any smaller.

Jody and I dragged J ten blocks or so to Inverleith Park, across from the Royal Botanic Garden, where we'd been told there would be a good view. J had been fearful of fireworks before, including that time in Boston when she had to cry before we listened, but she was nearly eight now, and we wanted to see the show and celebrate our last night in Scotland. Given the crowd we soon found ourselves in, Inverleith Park was well known as a good viewing ground. Trust us, we told J, this will be a good memory. Trust us.

Other than finding a place to sit, the size of the crowd in Inverleith Park didn't bother me. This would be one of the last times for a long time that being in a crowd wouldn't bother me. J kept complaining about the midges, that they were biting her ankles and making her itchy. There were no midges I could see or feel, and I'm a bug's first option. Those little dark bumps around her ankles were nothing to worry about, I assured J and myself in the same breath—maybe a rash from the virus she'd caught just as we left for Scotland. Coxsackie can leave a rash. I knew that much. Not a big deal.

I was glad the trip was ending, that we'd be on a plane home in the morning. I'd been to the land where McLean blood had been spilled over the centuries, in causes good, bad and in between. Mel Gibson made *Braveheart* on the blood of so many McLeans. My daughter left some of her own on an Edinburgh bus. I cleaned it up as best I could.

Funny thing is, the Scots weren't thrifty with their fireworks. They were extravagant, and the show went on for quite some time, the gothic outline of Edinburgh Castle illuminated with each new explosion. What a stirring conclusion to a life's dream, a visit to my ancestral homeland with my wife and daughter. My own flesh and blood.

Walking back to our apartment, I was sorry my sister hadn't come along. She'd planned to, made extensive arrangements for Mom's care, but cancelled when she was diagnosed with cancer. She apologized that cancer interfered with our plans. My sister is like that.

The idea had been to take her with us in thanks for caring for my parents in their latter years. Dad died six years before, and Mom had survived him so much longer than we expected. Mary Jo had done so much; teaching public school kids music by day, caring for elderly parents by night. The trip would be paid for in large part with money inherited from our dad's childless brother.

But there was no delaying the surgery, and my sister's trip to Scotland would have to wait. J and I managed a quick trip to Northern California to see Mary Jo and Mom before the surgery. I watched J bend down, kiss my mom tenderly, and tell her she loved her. I imagine I did something similar.

We returned home and prepared for a trip to a friend's wedding, and then on to Scotland. In between, we managed dinner with one branch of Jody's hybrid family. The conversation came round to elderly parents; Jody's stepmom's mother, J's only great grandmother, was failing. Someone said how wrenching it can be when a person outlives their own presence, and that maybe death is preferable. I'd thought the same thing before, when it wasn't personal, but now I heard an insensitive bluntness, and took offense but held my tongue. J took no offense but disagreed. She said she wanted my mom to live a lot longer, regardless of her condition. *I don't see her often,* my daughter said. *I want to be able to see her.*

Days later, my brother called to say Mary Jo's surgery had gone well, the surgeon felt he'd gotten all the cancer. But his tone said there was something else. Protective as ever, he wanted to reassure me that Mary Jo was recovering before he added, *Mom has passed away.*

I hate the term *passed away.* E.B. White taught me to hate it. The person died. Don't euphemize it. There's no softening this blow. Mom didn't pass away. She didn't go to a better place. She died. But I saved that lecture for another time.

Jody said we'd all go for the funeral, but that would mean missing a dear friend's wedding in New York State, in which Jody was a bridesmaid and J the flower girl. I argued that I should go to Mom's funeral, they should go to the wedding; that we'd all go to California again soon to reunite with my siblings. Jody was adamant, then anguished, but she finally agreed.

I wrote a eulogy on the plane to California. I had long before distanced myself from Mom's form of Catholicism, which to my perception she practiced with eyes closed to this world and open only to the next, but the good I continued to carry from her faith stemmed from its focus on the redemptive power of forgiveness, and I said so in her eulogy. Rosary on Sunday, funeral on Monday, red-eye back on Tuesday, arriving in Boston early Wednesday morning. We returned to Logan Airport that night for our flight to Edinburgh. We invited Jody's mom to replace my sister and join us for the first ten days of our trip, and she agreed.

J returned from the wedding with a sore throat, and her pediatrician, knowing we would soon be boarding a plane, quick-tested for strep. We wouldn't know definitively till we were in Scotland. He wrote a prescription for antibiotics just in case. When the strep test came back negative, we were relieved. We'd see Glasgow, my grandmother's birthplace; experience Highland Games on the Isle of Bute and the ancestral castle on Mull; hike through a rhododendron forest in Torridon; survey North Sea tide pools and attend a ceillidh in Nairn, where I watched my mother-in-law tear up at the beauty of the music and the authenticity of the gathering, just as my sister would have done.

We laughed loudly as we drove along the wrong side of the road listening to *George's Marvelous Medicine* on CD—*I've got bangers in my bottom!*—and discovered that Killiecrankie was not just another despicable and opportunistic Roald Dahl parent but a town en route to Saint Andrews from the Highlands.

We concluded our Scottish adventure in Edinburgh, after Jody's mom had returned to the States, and following a side trip to the ancient burial grounds at Clava Cairns, where I reflected on my mom's recent burial, and J—fed up with touring rock piles and hearing me drone on about ancestry—muttered in reply: *Obladi, oblada, life goes on, bra!* Sarcasm, too, is in the McLean blood.

In Edinburgh, Jody participated in a psychological conference, presenting a paper on the impact of siblings on issues later in life. J had no siblings to cause problems or offer solutions now or later. She and I adventured around the town where Harry Potter was created, riding daily in the front of double-decker buses. We didn't care where we went. We'd head toward Leith and the firth one day, east or south with no destination in mind the next. Walking through Leith Links, where Old Tom and Young Tom once competed but where stands no golf course now, just sporting fields, parkland and a playground, a young mother complained and shook a used hypodermic needle that had been abandoned on the grass where her child had been at play.

Back aboard a double-decker, J sat and waited until we'd come to a stop, then crawled around the filthy floor collecting as many discarded bus passes as she could before we started moving again. She gathered quite a wad, forming a collection treasured for a moment. We made funny faces into the double mirror that provided the driver down below a distorted view of the upper deck. Slowing to a stop with a car before us, it looked as though the bus was devouring the car: *chomp, chomp, chomp,* we said.

A young mother, her babe in arms and a prodigiously snotty-nosed toddler sat across from us. I have no other memory involving a stranger's child and snot, so why does this one stay with me? If I had heard of Purell at the time, less than a week before we descended into immunological hell, it wasn't on my shopping list.

Riding high and being together was what we craved. One day we headed west to the Edinburgh Zoo, which J already had seen with Jody as I played golf at Gullane, damn near rolling in that eagle putt with nobody watching. But she wanted to return to the zoo with me. I'd no idea there were so many varieties of penguin, and we got right up close as they pooped and splashed and waddled around in their infectious wonderland.

J was reluctant to walk all the way to the top of the zoo, which rises to one of the highest points in the city, but I wanted to see the elevated view, to look into the horizon in the distance on a clear and warm day. J complained, but the view was worth it, for a moment. Then J sat on a bench and her nose began to bleed.

The bleeding didn't stop right away. I wasn't sure what to do, although experience told me nose bleeds are no emergency. I had her sit back and hold my white handkerchief to her nose while I pinched. The bleeding slowed, then started up again. A tram delivered other zoo visitors to our elevated perch, and the driver offered us a ride to the bottom. We got water, and she drank and continued to hold my now red handkerchief to her nose. The bleeding became a trickle, stopped, and we exited the zoo and headed for the bus. J insisted on the upper level. The bleeding renewed but then slowed and finally ceased as we rode the bus. I'd say it lasted fifteen minutes; J says it was longer, and her memory tends to be less revisionist than mine.

We cut our day short, returned to our apartment, rested awhile, and J felt better. She got sick later that night, which I've come to attribute to my having her tilt her head back. You're not supposed to do that. I know that now. What you do is, you tip the head forward as you pinch the soft part of the nose, between the tip and the bony bridge, making certain to keep the head above the heart to slow the flow. Don't let go for five minutes, and if it continues to bleed, hold for another ten minutes. Ice helps. When it stops, take it easy for a while. All of this assumes you have platelets. If not, all bets are off. Within days I'd learn that J lacked enough platelets for a decent clot.

I've heard that some parents keep Roald Dahl's stories away from their kids. They're too dark. Dahl's adults are such idiots, weasels, inhuman brutes. Maybe I don't take such things seriously enough as a parent, and perhaps I ought to shelter my daughter from such characters, fictional or real. But I couldn't shelter my daughter from a darker reality than Roald Dahl ever conjured, although he seemed to see into our future in *George's Marvelous Medicine*. We listened to actor Richard E. Grant's reading on the road through Killiecrankie, and we howled at George in the kitchen deviously mixing a mad scientist's vile potion to give his Grandma a dose of her own: poisons and toxins and stinging, stinking fluids, crushed bones and blended bugs, the creepy crawly as curative. *If you only knew,* George says, *what I have in store for you.*

Soon doctors would tell my daughter the zoo was off limits indefinitely. Meanwhile they would give her bear bile, rabbit and horse serum, and regularly inject heparin, an anticoagulant derived from cows and pigs, into catheters surgically implanted on either side of her chest.

Jay McLean was a medical student when he discovered heparin. His bovine or porcine fluid, which he first found in dogs, would flow into my daughter's chest daily, serving to keep her life line flowing. Which meant at least one McLean-related product was serving a useful purpose within J's veins. Certainly McLean blood was no longer doing her any good. With 80-some transfusions over eight months, who knows whose blood was flowing through her.

I never met Jay McLean, but I communicated by email with his granddaughter after she introduced herself to the clan on Maclean.net and introduced me to heparin's McLean connection. It was comforting, I told her, to think that someone named McLean was giving my daughter a fighting chance. Then again, I'm not sure what blood line means anymore. My own flesh and blood isn't my own blood now. Since the bone marrow transplant, she has a stranger's blood and a whole new clan. For all I know, she has her own castle in the horizon in the distance. With luck, and darkly curative potions only Roald Dahl could mix, we'll visit it one day. She'll sign the clan book. I'll be just visiting.

CHAPTER TWO

A Port in a Storm

I learned of the funeral by email. We were days into a six-week stay on the Hematology/Oncology Ward at Boston Children's Hospital. J's illness was "life-threatening," they said, and my wife and I struggled to understand what that meant. Our understanding was not the same. Jody somehow separated the rational from the emotional. I heard life-threatening as weighing heavily toward fatal. I was frozen in shock, and unable to comprehend. I felt useless.

A friend's daughter had died in her twenties of cancer. The memorial service was at our neighborhood church, a mile or so from the hospital. I knew the father and the step-mother well, and felt compelled to attend. Jody was furious, said I was crazy, and I had no rebuttal. She knew my despair needed no encouragement. But attending didn't feel optional. I didn't know the young woman, only many of the broken hearts she'd left behind. I don't know why I was compelled to attend. Maybe it was a morbid curiosity, to gain and store away insight into what it's like for a father to mourn a daughter. Maybe I hadn't grieved my mom sufficiently after her death weeks earlier. I wanted the dad and stepmom to know I was there, out of some vague idea it would matter that I'd left my own daughter at the hospital to come and say goodbye to theirs. Maybe I craved context. But rationalizing is a waste of time. I just had to go.

At the funeral, I was asked about J's illness and described a playdate interrupted by bruises that served as my slap in the face and got me to take her to the doctor. Not waiting to be jolted awake would have been a good thing for all concerned, J in particular, but that's not the way it happened. While rereading notes from the time and reliving the awakening, and the frightful weeks that followed, I would shut down mid-story, losing my place in a verbal telling or nodding off mid-sentence at the keyboard, and coming to without a clue what the next word ought to be or how I got to the last one. This happened several times. I wore blinders through the worst of J's illness and treatment, and they served a useful purpose. Taking them off wasn't simple.

Early signs something was amiss ranged from the dark bumps I came to know as petechiea to the pronounced paleness of her beautiful skin, but J had always been light skinned and these seeming facts of the everyday didn't call out to me for immediate attention. If they did, I wasn't listening. Pimples, I told myself; that's what the bumps were. Concern about a fever that persisted well into our Scotland trip was tempered by good appetite and energy, while ibuprofen and acetaminophen masked what we asked. Take a pill, buck up, get on with discovering a blood line. Ibuprofen's blood-thinning properties have haunted me ever since.

I could see a pattern only in retrospect, when it was of no particular use other than as paternal penance. I'm ashamed of my slow awakening to the reality of J's physical decline, for assuming time and her own body would heal whatever was amiss. J delivered the wake-up call, through her cousin Emily. Two days after our return from Scotland, and a day before the school year was to begin, J and Emily joined me at the war zone that was our home, a late-1950s ranch-style box that was four months into renovation and another four months from becoming livable. Jody and I envisioned the renovated home as a social place to gather and nurture community, and not badger guests about symptoms or whether they'd wiped their feet.

As I tended to matters in the house, peering through spaces where walls once stood, the two cousins ran across the street to play. In a small, narrow yard, neighbors had created a magical habitat, complete with lush foliage and pond, and they invited J to make it her own. She did not hesitate, and watched toads grow from eggs, found salamanders hiding under bark, laughed loudly at frogs latched onto her wrist, providing lessons in the passions of mating season, when they would chirp their love songs in loud bursts heard a block away. In making myriad other discoveries in that blessed water, J came not simply to love nature but to feel a part of it. Soon that idyllic space would become a Superfund site for the immune-abandoned, just as J's friends were transformed, Jeckyl and Hyde-like, into sneezing, coughing monsters. Soon everyone and everything would pose risk.

Emily approached me in the driveway. She said J had large bruises and was scared. I went to J at the pond, and in that moment any claim to protective abilities drained from me with the swiftness that platelets were disappearing inside her body. We drove to the pediatrician. He was unavailable, but a colleague saw J, took me aside and said to take her directly to Children's Hospital. She didn't want to frighten me, and didn't call for an ambulance, but said J needed to be seen and assessed immediately in the emergency room. Emily stayed with us in what was fast transitioning from play on a sunny September New England day to something darker.

In time, J would describe Emily as her guardian angel.

I put J on the cellphone with Jody as we drove to Children's. J was nervous and quiet but already exhibiting a bravery I would marvel at, and cherish. I came to count on that courage to bolster my own sapped spirit. The waiting room at Children's was uncrowded and we were expeditiously escorted into a private room. When you're a kid with no immune system, sitting in a room full of fevers, coughs and retches is against doctor's orders. In our private room, J received her first of countless IV sticks. She still recalls the first, and the dread was magnified with each successive poke. Her first blood draw showed her platelet count to be low.

I didn't know how many platelets one human requires to function – a quarter million is a good, safe number—or that they could be counted. My education in blood of the literal, non-metaphorical type had begun. J was given a bag – of platelets, I think, or gamma globulin to stimulate platelet production—and diagnosed: ITP, or idiopathic thrombocytopenic purpura. The phrase meant nothing to me, and as a diagnosis had a lifespan shorter than a lymphocyte's, though part of it would follow us for months (the suffix –*penic*, meaning a deficiency), part of it forever (idiopathic). And yet, given the frightening physical symptoms of the revolt within J's body, and despite the fact that idiopathic means even the doctor doesn't know why this is happening, ITP was a somehow comforting diagnosis. Often the body takes care of the problem without explanation and returns to business as usual. ITP can be a mere blip on the timeline.

The head of the Emergency Department saw J's name on a chart and came to us. Dr. Michael Shannon was a friend, a neighbor, a wise and calming presence. He explained ITP in a way that we could at least begin to comprehend. And after a long and traumatic day and evening at Children's, he sent us home. Michael knew we could return in minutes. He said to keep J from activities likely to cause bruises, and to follow up with her pediatrician early the next week, when it was hoped that another blood draw would reveal her system was righting itself. J had not nearly enough sleep to attend her first day of school, so we kept her home. Home was in the basement at my in-laws, who four months earlier had welcomed us for however long our renovation would last. Their generosity was without limit.

After a quietly recuperative day, J joined her classmates for what would be her only day of second grade. We explained the situation to Libby, her teacher, and asked that J be withheld from physical activities. The day went uneventfully, and Libby thought to take J's picture to post with the other class members on a wall by the entryway. In it, her long, straight hair surrounds a pale, thin but sweetly smiling face. It is a photo that makes me wonder where my awareness was. In the next photo posted outside that same classroom, J would be bald, and still smiling sweetly.

On Sunday, the three of us attended church. It was Opening Sunday, a reunion after summer vacations, and launched a new ministry. I had spent two years on a search committee that brought co-ministers to our church. I had so much confidence in the ministers. I looked forward to seeing the congregation grow with these deeply spiritual guides. I hadn't anticipated needing their pastoral gifts right away myself.

That afternoon, a family from J's school hosted a gathering. As Jody and I described the events of the week to concerned friends, J found the exuberant play of the other children irresistible, and joined in. I cautioned her to take it easy, to avoid rough play, and she complied while managing to run a bit and have some fun. It was sticky hot that day, and later, back at my in-laws' home, we cranked up the air conditioners. J got to bed early in preparation for the school week, and when I checked in on her she'd kicked her covers off and looked cold to me. I covered her up and tried not to wake her, but she looked up briefly, then closed her eyes, snuggled under her covers and gave me a thankful grin. It was a familiar grin, one reserved for being noticed and tucked in after she'd kicked off her covers. Sometimes I thought she kicked them off on purpose so I'd have to cover her up. Sometimes it was accompanied by a *Thanks, Pop.* It warmed me every time. The memory warms me still.

Jody woke me up. J's nose was bleeding and she had a fever. Back at Children's Hospital Emergency, cauterizing stopped the bloody nose. Nothing would stop the fever, not for long and not for weeks. Another painful IV stick into her thin arm. Not only platelets were fast disappearing. Her red cell count also was low, as was her white count. A new word: neutrophils – stem cells, baby whites. When they're low, you're not making enough white cells. As a diagnosis, ITP also was disappearing.

There would be no sending her home now, no entrusting her to the attentive inadequacy of her parents. J's entire blood supply was crashing, except perhaps for the T lymphocytes, the killer cells; the mother fuckers. If you have an infection, you want T cells on your side. They do a number on certain cancers. But they can become confused and attack what is not foreign at all. They are soldiers on your side one moment, inexplicably Al Qaeda the next. Anarchists. *Are you with us or against us?* T cells, it seems, can be both.

J was admitted to Seven West that night. The late, great Seven West. The hematology/oncology wing at Boston Children's Hospital has since moved to another floor, another direction, but Seven West will live forever as the place I go when chaos descends. Seven West is my middle-aged blankie. It is where unbelievable bad news was delivered (*her bone marrow appears dead*); where newly bald kids were in the majority, their hair clogging the communal tub; where everyone was more or less in the same boat, though some were destined to stay onboard longer; where J became expert at Ms. Pac-Man and taught it to the head of Emergency; where we began to learn that paranoia cannot always rule and sometimes it's a good thing to take a kid without platelets for a joy ride on her IV pole.

Brooke took charge, and immediately became a source of comfort, compassion and understanding. There were other nurses to come, hundreds, some Brooke's equal; no one was better. We looked to Brooke to make sense of our overturned world. Other nurses attained a similar

21

elevated place—Suzanne, who let J soak her in the shower; Jenn, with a different and festive set of scrubs for every day; Phaedra, for that wonderfully goofy dance. Each could put J at ease even as they inflicted unpleasant treatment upon her.

But Brooke, because she was so smart, because she was there from the start, because of the way she "got" J immediately, achieved mythic stature. She explained things well, and patiently, and we listened to her closely. Jody or I must have asked her whether something in the fluctuation in J's blood counts was considered "normal." We were trying to understand, trying to bring order to the chaos, trying to find someone who would say, *If you do this, everything will be all right.* There was no one to say that. Instead, Brooke smiled her wonderful and deeply empathic smile. She might have sighed; who knows where a Heme-Onc nurse's emotions go to hide? She couldn't tell us where this adventure was headed, how long it would last, what would be the same when we emerged on the other side and what would be forever changed. She could only say, *This is a new normal.*

In the new normal, fevers don't go away for weeks, doctors can't explain why, and though they'd load J with antibiotics, antivirals and antifungals in scattershot hunt for the cause, they'd disagree on Tylenol. The pediatric attending wanted to give Tylenol to bring the fever down and comfort J. Doctors from Hematology/Oncology and Infectious Diseases did not. Masking the fever could make it harder to find the cause, and the fever's cause might well be related to the collapse of J's immune system, perhaps even to its resurrection. They didn't want to mess with the road map, but the road map was reading 102-plus. J was burning up, and whether or not she could have Tylenol to cool her down depended on which doctor from which department had been through our room last, and which nurse knew which doctor to listen to. Is it more compassionate to make a kid feel better or to find out what's threatening her life? First do no harm. Sounds good on paper.

In the new normal, you're confined to a small room shared with another pediatric patient, separated by a curtain. Each side has a TV, and with luck your roommate won't watch in the wee hours, or if she does, it won't be total trash, and if it is total trash, the volume will be at a reasonable level. With luck, your roommate isn't a chemo-cranky infant who can't sleep.

In the new normal, the neighbor kids are bald. J had one of the only full heads of hair on Seven West, where most were being treated for one cancer or another. In the new normal, shampoo with conditioner is quaint. In the new normal, if you beat the cleaning crew to the communal bath, you see your future in large clumps of another child's hair. J still needed shampoo. It felt like a blessing and a privilege.

In the new normal, the newspaper says there's a war in Iraq, genocide in Sudan, American civil liberties are becoming something for history books, should we ever get J back to school, and I couldn't give a damn. It's 3 in the morning, J is finally getting some sleep, and the sweet infant on the other side of the curtain, with tumors amounting to no insignificant percentage of her total body weight, has begun to retch and wail loudly, from the chemo, I suspect. The only thing that will soothe her is a CD of new age lullabies. It amounts to "Turaluralura" sung over and over by Teletubbies. Incessant meets insipid. J is frustrated. *I can't sleep,* she says. Do I ask the other parent to turn the music down, preferably off, when that seems to be the only thing distracting their absolute angel from her pain and keeping her from shrieking even more? There are no private rooms on Seven West, unless you're infectious and quarantined, lucky you, or terminal. Do I ask the nurse to switch rooms? I tried that, but even when possible, doesn't that just make Teletubby "Turaluralura" some other chemo'd-up kid's problem?

Meanwhile J couldn't have Tylenol for her fever, hadn't slept because doctors or nurses kept coming in to check on her or her roommate, and hadn't eaten because she was NPO, short for nothing per oral but which means you starve until the surgeon or radiologist gets around to you. If they don't get around to you, you can have something to eat, then be NPO again tomorrow while they try to fit you in.

There is a strange competition set off between families with children who have life-threatening illnesses. Shared rooms are no way to heal. But then, if you made them all private rooms, there'd be no place for half the kids, and the place is full up as it is. New arrivals get sent to another floor, where the nurses are great but don't specialize in cancer or blood disorders, and where the kid next door has a good, strong immune system and a nasty case of strep. In the new normal, the hospital is where the experts and meds and bags of blood are, but it feels like no place to get well.

In the new normal, you find out who your friends are. If you're lucky, you have a lot of them. We were lucky. People wanted to cook for us, bring us books and CDs and videos, house and feed the cat and guinea pigs, decide which light fixtures or sinks to put in our renovated home, and try to respect the wall our prescribed isolation had erected and yet somehow scale it and deliver some solace."

In the new normal, I got sick of answering the compassionately asked question, "What do you need?" *I need a fucking immune system for my kid!* I never actually said that, but I wanted to. I wanted to bite someone, but who? No one was at fault. Not even God. I'm a Unitarian, so even the Almighty got off the hook. But the compassion, concern and empathy of friends were wearying me. I needed them—we needed them, we valued them—but only when the time was right. How do you manage that?

Jody's sister Kristin became our buffer, our scheduler, and someone to relieve J of "boring" hours with me. Kristin set up a blog through the organization Carepages and it quickly became an invaluable resource for Jody and I, helped to transcend our isolation, gave us a place to go with our hopes and fears, and allowed family and friends near and far to follow our progress. Kristin posted the first message on Sept. 20, 2005, early in J's hospitalization: *J was full of lots of laughs today when I visited her. She still has a slight fever which they are working on reducing so they can begin the drug therapies which will hopefully get her bone marrow working again. She is moving into a private room to get a bit more peace and quiet. Since it was such a visitor party last week, Paul and Jody are really restricting visitors at this time.*

A private room. Must've been a slow week for new kids with cancer.

The Carepage gave us control of the information flow. Jody and I craved knowing what was going on among family local and distant, among school friends, church friends, friends of friends as far away as Switzerland. When Jody or I would update someone before we had the blog, in our confusion or sleepless state we'd provide incomplete information or they'd mishear, and soon we'd hear back from someone else who'd been confused or misinformed along the grapevine. You simply can't tell someone you're on Heme/Onc and not have it come out "cancer." I hated my repeated reply, *No, it's not a cancer.* I was glad it wasn't cancer. But people understand cancer on some level, so they understand the seriousness. When it's not cancer, there's a certain relief. But what relief is it, really, to know that whatever it is that is not cancer still might very well kill your daughter? There were no leukemia cells in J's blood, and thank God for that. There wasn't much of anything in her blood. J's first bone marrow biopsy showed that. It was conducted by Heme/Onc fellow Jennifer Whangbo. She would become the doctor with us most closely and consistently.

Subsequent days and weeks were a blur of pediatricians, infectious disease specialists, hematologists, oncologists, bone marrow specialists, chaplains. As a rule, they'd arrive just when the chemo'd up infant in the bed next to us stopped wailing, Teletubby "Turaluralura" was silenced, and we'd finally fallen asleep.

Cable news was reporting regularly on the aftermath of Hurricane Katrina. The first I heard of Katrina, I was standing in queue before sunrise at the starter's shack at Saint Andrews. I was fifth in line behind four "oil bidness" buddies from Texas and Louisiana. The hurricane hadn't hit yet, and one of them was animatedly cussing out his brother-in-law for stubbornly refusing to evacuate. The guy's sister and her kids got out, but the brother-in-law was a hard ass, and the sister couldn't reach him. I wondered about him as J slept and I watched the despair and chaos on the TV in our room on Seven West. The sound was down. Images were enough.

J's blood counts showed critically low levels of white cells, neutrophils, platelets and red cells, and a bone marrow aspiration led to diagnosis of a rare and poorly understood disease that at least gave us something to work with: aplastic anemia. The diagnosis gained an adjective: severe. Aplastic anemia is something of a catch-all for when a person's bone marrow ceases production of blood. It occurs to only one or two in a million, though that number is bound to change as science better understands the disease and its causes, which can be genetic, viral, bacterial or environmental. It doesn't have a particular age bias, and it can be reversible; that is, a body sometimes can be convinced to go back into production and not count on transfusions for survival.

I posted on the CarePage: *J is in remarkably good spirits. My brother called yesterday from Southern California, and told me how hard our news had hit him. I put him on the phone with J and she cheered him up. She's magic that way.*

Neutropenia means if you get sick, your body can't do a damn thing about it because production of baby white cells has shut down. You can't go near anyone who might be infectious, and yet you're in the hospital, where most everyone's infectious, except on Seven West, where most every patient is neutropenic. *Paging Dr. Heller, Dr. Joseph Heller.* There isn't a patient on the entire ward with an immune system worth a damn, and staff and visitors know this and behave accordingly. A roommate's sister had a bad case of the sniffles. Wary, I parted the curtain and checked. She was sobbing. Sobbing is contagious, but not in the concerning way.

The doctors told J a few things were off the menu, notably popcorn and Doritos, foods that cut the gums. The mouth, it turns out, is a dangerous thing to have when you're immune compromised. And yet, nasty and infectious as the mouth may be, J couldn't brush her teeth, which might cause bleeding and stir up bacteria. She was given sponge sticks and a special mouthwash. Her mouth was quarantined from her body.

J's fever spiked to 104. Broad antibiotics didn't resolve the problem and she was given the antifungal drug ambizome, a name we'd repeat many times when doctors would ask, *Any allergies?* With ambizome, you watch for side effects, especially kidney function. It gave J a rash. Infectious Diseases believed the fevers had a viral cause, though the belief wasn't enough to preclude taking the antifungal just in case. New word: aspergillus. A fungus, we were told, would wreak havoc and must be avoided. Antibiotics were needed, too, because a bacterial infection could run rampant in a body with no defense. Lacking knowledge of the cause, J was treated for everything it might be. Throw darts by the handful and see what hits the board.

J's rash appeared within minutes of the first dose of ambizome, but Pediatrics recalled seeing the rash during morning rounds, before the ambizome. I didn't remember it that way. Infectious Diseases didn't remember it that way, either. But before we could sort it out, we learned that even though J likely did not suffer from an infectious disease, the fact she was being treated by Infectious Diseases meant isolation. So she couldn't leave her room, and for the first time in days she felt like getting out of bed and touring around a bit. *Sorry, honey.*

Before long, Pediatrics lost the vote, the rash was attributed to ambizome, and J stopped taking it. Infectious Diseases still suspected the fevers had a viral cause, but we couldn't count on that. Another antifungal was prescribed. A relative suggested that taking so many antibiotics, antifungals and anti-whatnots couldn't be good for a body in the long run. I laughed a pissed-off laugh. Oh, to be able to think in terms of the long run. To be able to see that far into the future, and not just to the next bag of blood, tapped from some anonymous being like syrup from a maple. Whatever the cause, we needed the fevers to stop, so we could get on with treating J's disease.

The urgency of moving forward with treatment was delivered by Akiko Shimamura, a hematologist uniquely gifted with both adults and children who was involved in J's care nearly from the start. Dr. Shimamura understood bone marrow disease like few others, and she would become an important voice to us. If this illness had to happen, thank God it happened a short walk from Akiko's place of business and in a time when such a healer could rise to such a level of understanding. She said the medical attempt to right J's immune system would last four days, begin within a week of the fever abating, and would combine cyclosporine and antithymocyte globulin, or ATG. Both work by suppressing the immune system. I did not readily comprehend the idea of suppressing to restore, but my comprehension wasn't required, only a leap of faith.

Jody and I heard stories of parents separated from their neutropenic kids. Those days were over. We wouldn't be separated from J, unless we became sick ourselves. If there was something fortunate about J's illness, it was that it came in a time when isolation wasn't a bubble. With a life-threatening illness, timing is everything.

Family and friends called with diagnoses: We'd been in Martha's Vineyard over the summer, perhaps the illness had a tick-borne origin. Could it have been toxic dust kicked up during renovation? J had spent hours with my sister's birds in August, and one of them died that fall. West Nile?

Was it her guinea pigs? Doctors ran every test they could think of. The desire to answer why was widely shared but soon abandoned.

The church was packed for the memorial. A minister I'd gotten to know during our congregation's search spoke eloquently and humanly of the young woman.

I sat toward the back. Teachers from J's school, including the stepmom in mourning, were well aware of our situation and surprised to see me there. *Talk to Jody about that,* I said with a smirk.

From many stories emerged a remarkable life. They made me wish I'd known the young woman. She was by all accounts brilliant, compassionate and made others' lives better, and now she was gone, leaving parents to absorb the unfairness and somehow carry on. I watched friends, teachers, the minister and the stepmom remember her movingly. No one suggested she'd gone to a better place. I wondered what it would be like to attend my own daughter's funeral. Would I have the courage to speak? I would want to. I would have to. But could I?

Sitting in the pew, awash in the expressions of love for a young woman who had died and of caring and compassion for the parents left grieving, I began an accounting of all the things I loved in my daughter – her smile, her kindness, her sense of humor, her emerging musical gifts, her spirit, her hugs—and I found there was always one more thing I'd overlooked. Which made me think of a Monty Python routine, *Nobody expects the Spanish Inquisition,* in which the robed and hilariously accented Python, to his frustration, keeps remembering one more weapon. *Our weapon is surprise. Surprise and fear. Are two weapons.* I laughed to myself, and hoped no one noticed.

Wrong time to laugh, totally wrong. Like when I was an altar boy at a funeral, standing beside Monsignor Murphy and choking on the incense smoke and knowing that making eye contact with my friend on the other side of the monsignor was going to do me in, but then we made eye contact, and struggled mightily not to laugh before the grieving family of strangers.

But what better way to think of my daughter, my still alive daughter, than with something that made me laugh? There was always something else to love about J. That list would never be complete. Now there was another: In a dark and sober moment, she made me think of an old Monty Python routine. *Amongst our weapons are such elements as...*

In laughing to myself I enraged myself and wondered, what sort of mind composes his daughter's eulogy while she's alive? A perverse mind, I suppose, confused and overwhelmed and a month removed from eulogizing my own mother and remembering her sustaining faith as one grounded in forgiveness and redemption. Perhaps I would have had such morbid thoughts even without close proximity to my mother's death, but when I first heard the phrase *life-threatening illness*, my mind went immediately to death. I didn't assume my daughter was going to die, but the collapse of her body came so suddenly, so unexpectedly and mysteriously, that I couldn't explain it, and I roiled with desire for a rational understanding that I knew would never come. I felt sorry for myself, a middle-aged man with but one child, and perhaps destined to outlive that one child.

I broke down a number of times—by myself, on the phone with a brother, in conversation with Jody's stepmom, Lucy, who was about to bury her own mother, and who meanwhile was working the phones and Web to better understand the gravity of her granddaughter's illness. At the same time, a friend of Lucy's committed suicide. Lucy is perhaps the most resourceful person I've ever known. That her resourcefulness could somehow survive and transcend the chaos swirling around her was beyond my comprehension, but I studied it. It became a model.

I walked out of the funeral with a heightened awareness my friends' daughter was dead and mine was alive; that their daughter had touched many and lived profound moments that would remain sacred in the hearts of friends and family, and that my daughter had lives yet to touch, moments yet to be sanctified.

I left knowing the distinction between a coffin's clarity and the ambiguity of a hospital room. I came away understanding the space between fatal and life-threatening. You can fit a lot of hope into that space.

I walked back to the hospital, where my daughter was alive.

I posted to J's friends, *If you think your Math homework is hard, try counting platelets and hemaglobins and neutrophils!* Someone emailed that I shouldn't try to cheer people up. I hit reply, typed *Fuck off*, then hit cancel instead of send. I still had some judgment left.

Jody and I met to discuss diagnosis and treatment with Drs. Shimamura and Whangbo in the room where I'd slept. Small, dimly lit, with a window not to the outdoors but to a Heme/Onc hallway, and a sofa that reconfigured into a single bed occupied most nights by the odd parent out, the room served many purposes. Nursing staff used it to prepare parents for outpatient plans or other eventualities; social workers to connect parents in support groups; doctors to deliver verdicts, best guesses and to map paths forward; families to discuss options, or close the door and cry.

Dr. Whangbo, direct, measured and a reliable source of a compassionate smile and a thoughtful explanation, arrived first and explained J's bone marrow aspiration. They'd found no leukemia, which was a relief. They'd also found so little else of what a body needs to survive: red cells to deliver oxygen, platelets to stop the bleeding, white cells to fight infections. Seeking support and insight, Jody and I invited Dr. Shannon, our friend, and Dr. George Daly, a colleague of a friend of Lucy's. He knew Dr. Shimamura well and stem cells even better. Only days before, there had been hope that time and J's own body might collaborate to correct her problem. But a week into her Seven West stay, the diagnosis had become severe aplastic anemia. It was time for Jody and I to comprehend what we could, and to act.

The others arrived and crowded in. My hair wasn't combed and my teeth weren't brushed. I remember a doctor using the word "dead" to describe J's bone marrow. Jody does not recall this, which makes me suspect it was never said at all. And yet I remember it.

Dr. Daly opened my eyes to the wonder of stem cells and helped me see the possibilities amid the risks. Fear and hope, in one untidy package.

I met separately with the ahead of pediatric transplant at Children's and Dana-Farber Cancer Institute. Transplant was far off, last-ditch, but Jody and I needed to understand it and prepare for the possibility. I left the meeting glad to have such a brilliant mind involved in my daughter's care, awed by her comprehension of all that went into a successful transplant, and frightened by my inability to grasp a word of it. My notes could be written in sanskrit.

Slowly our challenge was sinking in. Slowly wasn't fast enough.

The immune-suppressing ATG and cyclosporine posed less risk than transplant and held great promise to generate a full, positive response in J within six months. According to the literature, it did so in 70 percent of cases. And yet a full and positive response meant independence from transfusions; it did not mean cure. Only transplant offered the potential for cure. The doctors knew we hadn't saved any cord blood from J's birth, so she couldn't be transplanted with her own stem cells. Saving them had never occurred to us, and yet in the few short years since J's birth, scientists had turned cord blood, so often lost to the cleanup crew, into lifesaving gold. Understanding of J's illness and ways to treat it was changing before our eyes.

Without cord blood, the next question was: *Does J have a sibling?* The answer was no, and another child was not in our plans. Neither had aplastic anemia been in our plans for the one child we did have. Jody and I would have to make this choice for J, and soon. Would we create a life for the initial purpose of harvesting bone marrow to save that child's sibling? There are scientific means of fertilizing an egg and assessing its DNA to improve the one-in-four odds of obtaining a marrow match. That level of understanding creates a sense of awe in me, as well as moral confusion over the manipulation of life. And yet transplants for aplastic anemia have a greater chance of curative success when performed within a year of the initial diagnosis.

There wasn't a lot of time to sit with this information. If we were to create a life for the initial purpose of saving J, how would that effect us as parents, as husband and wife; what would it mean long term for that new life, and for J? What if the transplant failed anyway? If we decided not to create that life, were we sacrificing J? The ethical considerations were more than I could process, and yet the bottom line was I would do anything to save my daughter. I would create another child, trust doctors to make the child a match for J, harvest the bone marrow, and love that child as though there were no gray in his or her reason for being.

Easy for me to say. I wasn't the one who would carry the child.

More immediately, a daunting and shape-shifting pile of daily meds needed to get inside of J. Some could be infused. Some came in liquid form. Some were pills, and it's asking a lot for a seven-year-old to knock down a collection of pills in a timely manner. Some angel suggested practicing with miniature M&Ms. J wasn't a quarter way through the first bag when she smiled at me and said, *This is easy!* And so it was.

Perhaps the wretched cyclosporine provided her incentive. Squirting the skunky goo into her mouth, swallowing it and keeping it down were difficult. Just putting it to her lips was difficult. And so it was a literally bitter irony that even after she'd learned to swallow pills, her doctors weren't willing to switch cyclosporine to capsule form until they'd found a consistent dose. But soon she willingly swallowed twenty-something pills daily. She'd give me a look – *again? already?* – followed by *Oh, whatever,* and down they'd go. Learning to swallow pills made hard realities so much easier.

And so, in time, did the port-a-cath. Not everything J needed could be delivered in pill form. Every day her courage bolstered my own, but her spirit sagged with each IV needle shoved into her. They hurt going in, they hurt staying in, and they hurt coming out, especially when the tape came off. There needed to be a better way to deliver all the fluids involved—the blood products, the serum, the sustenance when she couldn't eat. There were no good places to insert the IVs, only marginally less painful ones. They tended to kink or clog, requiring a new one and another poke. When they didn't kink or clog, they remained in place, taped to her arm, hand or foot, sometimes in two places at once. The tape would come off, and she'd be in tears. She came to anticipate the pain, and cry in advance when the IV was laid on a tray before her.

A roommate with cancer, an impish veteran of countless violations, had her catheter removed because it had been in for a month or so and had crossed the threshold from necessary evil to unacceptable risk. We listened from the other side of the curtain as a nurse poked about for a vein not already beaten into submission. One arm was accessed twice without any blood to show for the discomfort. After a series of muffled, deadened *ows,* the nurse moved on to the next arm, where there was success. The child sounded as deflated as her veins. Perhaps that muffled, deadened reaction comes from prolonged experience, but J, something of a newcomer, couldn't get used to the pokes. It's different for every kid.

Because of infection risk and the fact J would get accessed multiple times weekly for months, our attention was drawn to the port-a-cath. The device takes its name from "portal" and "catheter." A small reservoir, roughly the size of a short stack of quarters, is coated with a self-sealing silicone bubble. Because it is surgically implanted beneath the skin, which is allowed to heal over it, the infection risk is low, and the silicone can be punctured hundreds of times, perhaps a thousand, before a replacement is needed. A small bump on the chest appears as a light bruise. The skin can be numbed topically prior to accessing. This was all to the good.

The catch was, the port needed to be surgically installed, surgery meant bleeding, and bleeding needs platelets to stop. This was absurd to me. They knew she couldn't stop bleeding on her own, didn't hang onto transfused platelets for long, and yet these experts advised surgery?

Dr. Shannon, finished with his day's work in Emergency, stopped by to see how we were doing. I told him about the ongoing trauma of IV sticks, that we were being advised to have a port installed and that surgery made no sense to me. Dr. Shannon, whose calm was such that he once performed a spinal tap on his own son, understood my fear of surgery. He said this was manageable and that we would look back on the port as a vital and good choice for J. This was an important conversation for me. I trusted Michael fully. He knew and cared about J personally. His advice simplified the decision. We told the doctors to load her up with platelets and schedule the surgery, and they said they would, just as soon as the fevers abated.

J was in her hospital bed on the phone with Victoria. J and Victoria had been close friends for most of their lives. They discovered a shared love of critters. They invented games. They rolled around on our lawn with Heart and Flower, J's guinea pigs, fed them dandelion leaves, created a guinea pig circus. They played at Victoria's apartment with her mice, a community whose population seemed to expand with each playdate. J and Victoria hadn't seen each other in weeks and Victoria's parents said she was having a tough time getting her head around J's illness and absence. On the phone, the separation evaporated as if by magic. Victoria filled J in on the death of a rat belonging to another friend, Abigail, and I was struck at the ease with which they discussed death. J recalled feeling the rat's tumors. Abigail would soon adopt J's guinea pigs.

J loved her critters, and often asked if she could see them. Guinea pigs are prolific poopers, unpleasant in healthy times, deadly in times of neutropenia. Repeatedly the doctors told her no. No to guinea pigs. No to her cat. No to the toads in the garden. No to the new animals she dreamt up daily. J hated hearing it, but she kept asking. If yes was in her future, how would she know if she didn't keep asking?

Lucy returned from her mom's funeral outside Detroit. Lucy isn't a blood relation of J's, but their connection would be no more profound if they shared DNA. J and Lucy are soul mates of an intergenerational and timeless sort. While organizing and attending her mother's funeral, Lucy had been working the phones. She's connected. She has friends at the Whitehead Institute, at Harvard and Caltech, and they know stem cells or people who know stem cells. By phone from her dying mother's side, Lucy had asked my permission to make some calls. Between sobs, I said yes, please. Permission granted, she sheepishly admitted she'd already made a few. *Time is of the essence.* Thinking inside the box was no longer possible, advisable or remotely desirable.

Fevers continued to delay treatment with suppressants. It was urgent that we get on with that treatment, but the suppressants themselves would cause all kinds of problems, fevers for one, and to begin on top of an existing fever required a more desperate situation. That we weren't yet desperate enough was a comfort, of sorts. I discussed the port-a-cath with J. She hated the idea.

Our roommate was a loud one, and I'd become less conflicted about complaining. A room came open at midnight, but on Seven West, time of day was irrelevant. We moved a few doors down. J's new roommate was a Jimmy Fund kid with neuroblastoma who would throw out the first pitch at Fenway Park that night. I was jealous. Not about the first pitch. If the kid was going to Fenway, she must have neutrophils.

I called Jody's mother, Joan, to ask if we could move in for a while. We couldn't return to our gutted home yet, and the doctors were concerned about our returning to Gerry and Lucy's basement. There'd been so much rain throughout the summer, and the basement was damp. Damp was a problem—the neutropenia/aspergillus risk. Joan lived on the fifth floor of a century-old Back Bay apartment building, as dry as they come. The doctors also worried about dust, but Hepa air filters could take care of that. *Of course you can stay with me*, Joan said. We told Gerry and Lucy why, when J was at last released from Children's, we couldn't return to their home. They were understanding. They always are. But it hurt. It had to. It felt like slapping generosity in the face.

J's blood counts revealed little change. But as I learned to read them, I noticed something new with each new set. One day I noticed C for critical. The page was lousy with C's.

Doctors ordered an MRI, a chamber of horrors worthy of a Voldemort scene in Harry Potter. The MRI is both miracle machine and brute, pounding like a death metal band, pounding and pounding some more, with the kid strapped inside the coffinlike tube.

Radiology generally is a brutal department. J's mysteries demanded radiologists, but I couldn't return her to Seven West soon enough. The waiting room in Radiology was always full, but the specialty is machines and shadowy images, not people. J was frightened, shaking and needed to remain perfectly still for the chamber to do its work. Starved for the day, J was given nembutal to keep her absolutely still. Nembutal joined ambizome on the list of things to NEVER GIVE OUR DAUGHTER AGAIN. Afterward she saw double for 24 hours, which made it pretty much impossible to eat.

When she lost the double vision, but with a kinked and useless IV still taped to her foot and inflicting jolts of pain, J told her nurse that when she grew up she would invent a device to read blood and its contents externally. There will be no needle sticks. If this doesn't win her a Nobel Prize, it'll win her a standing O on Seven West. I know which is the higher honor.

J was, at best, tolerant of the blog. *Don't put that on the Carepage!*, she'd say. And yet the blog became invaluable to Jody and I as a place to process the day, to stay connected with our communities, to read messages of support from friends and family. J felt another area of control slipping away. Jody and I promised to respect her privacy in our postings while honoring the genuine interest in our plight. J and I talked a lot about it. I'm comfortable writing this story now because of those conversations. She's been through enough. I don't mean to put her through more.

Our home renovation proceeded largely without us. The architect and contractor were Jody's aunt and uncle. If they weren't handling the construction, work might have stopped. David and Linda's way of helping us was to make decisions when possible and simplify the ones we needed to make. I went to the house whenever I could, to see the progress, to hang out with David's crew, to envision J sleeping, peaceful and well, in her new bedroom. The visits were blessings, but it was a long time before I could return without remembering the day I awakened to the symptoms.

At 7:40 a.m., the cell phone of J's new roommate's mom rang to the electronic tune of "Dancing Queen." My fevered daughter and I awoke to Digital Abba. *If you're going through Hell, keep going.* Winston Churchill said that. It's on a card on a wall at my sister's house.

The MRI found a spot in J's brain, and required a second look. Brain surgery somehow entered the conversation for a kid who couldn't stop bleeding. The hematologists wanted to schedule a lumbar puncture immediately after the MRI so J wouldn't be sedated twice. Radiology wouldn't consider the idea. They had their reasons, apparently, but it seemed unfeeling and bureaucratic and my daughter was the loser. I was furious, being an asshole and coming to understand a patient's need for an advocate. Nurse Brooke, God bless her, intervened and beat her platelet-filled head against the wall that was Radiology. She got nowhere. J had another hard recovery from sedation, but the MRI brought good news: the spot in her brain was old blood, probably residual from the same platelet crash that required cauterizing a bloody nose. There was no sign of new bleeding. The lumbar puncture was cancelled. J could eat, just as soon as she stopped seeing double. She was not a happy kid.

Me to J on September 26 (no procedure): *I know you're not hungry, honey, but you've got to eat to keep up your strength.*

Me to J on September 27 and 28 (MRI, port surgery): *I know you're hungry, honey, but you can't eat today.*

If I get lucky, and J's problem is solved, I'll have to study up on eating disorders. Drinking disorders, too. But I digress.

I posted: *"J awoke today knowing she'd soon be heavily sedated and in the OR to have her "port" installed. As she was wheeled out of her room in Seven West, I asked her if she'd slept well. "I'm not sure," she said, grinning broadly, "but I'm GOING to!" Even on the way to the operating room, she cracks me up. Being prepped for OR, she received her first dose of "funny juice," and soon she was giggling. She said she saw two of Jody. She said she saw two of the anesthesiologist. She said she saw two of me. I asked how many chins I had. "Four," she replied.*

Badabing!"

J's anxiety about port surgery was eased by a 7-year-old roommate. She had her port for a year, and said it was a lot better than IV's and too many needle sticks. J euphemized surgery as a *procedure* and had an extra day to think about it because of some complication about which I'm ignorant and it's probably best that way. J got bumped. We found out after she'd been NPO all day. I wondered about a situation so dire for surgeons to postpone a child with a life-threatening illness. In sports, the losers say, *There's always tomorrow.* This isn't true, of course. There isn't always tomorrow. It's an optimistic way of viewing things, but it's not true.

A day later I wondered what life had been bumped by our own surgical complications.

J was wheeled in at 8 a.m. As I sat with her in pre-op, a boy across from us howled for his mom and dad, who were nowhere in sight. J asked why he was howling. I didn't know. I buried my head in *Junie B Jones,* read aloud and hoped Junie B could change the subject. I felt helpless to comfort J.

The surgeon was Rusty. That was his name, not his performance review. He had a very good reputation. And yet there's something ominous about having a surgeon wielding a sharp metal instrument, about to use it on your child, who's known as Rusty. The anesthesiologist was an idiot, with a specialty in dark humor inappropriate for a kid about have her chest cut open. He was better suited to embalming, and blessedly someone noticed and he was replaced by another who knew how to put a kid at ease. The replacement was charming and calming. He introduced J to propofol. She'll never forget him. She'll never remember him, either. Such is the beauty of propofol.

The port-a-cath was placed on the left side of J's chest, the catheter running under the surface of her skin and entering a major vein near her clavicle, feeding a tube two to three inches long that led down into the portal.

I sat in the waiting room with other parents. A couple I took to be Vietnamese sat across from me. The man said little, but stoically held the woman's hand as she sobbed. She sobbed for a long while. Anytime someone in scrubs walked past the window, we looked up expectantly. When their turn came, parents gathered themselves and went to their children. I buried my head in the *New York Times*. I read the same Thomas Friedman paragraph 10 times. Many surgeons in scrubs passed by before Rusty appeared in the window. He gave me the thumbs up, and said they'd come get me when J was ready.

Around 10, I met J in Recovery. The expectation was, once she'd recovered from the sedation, we'd return to Seven West, and put the port right to use with an ATG infusion. But at 10:20, J told me her side hurt, and soon had trouble breathing. They took an X-ray. In minutes, Propofol Man returned J to some distant place. Rusty apologized and got busy again with his sharp tools. The vein hadn't sealed around the port tube's entry point in her neck, and fluid leaked into her lung. Rusty loaded her with more platelets, inserted a drainage tube into her side, and she soon was back in Recovery.

Going into surgery, you're warned of complications. I kept reminding myself that J had a life-threatening illness little understood in spite of hearts and minds devoted to that understanding. Aplastic anemia affected maybe two in a million. When you're told that certain problems occur one percent of the time and your child's disease is two in a million, give or take, risk of one percent is little comfort. A nun prayed for J, perhaps *with* J, in the OR. I'm not sure what J made of this. Jesus was the nun's point of reference, the one she went to for intervention, comfort or both. Years earlier, thinking of what Jesus went through had helped me in difficulty of one sort or another, but not so much now. *Why have you abandoned me, father, o father?*

As the sedation wore off, J was in pain and my touch only added to her discomfort. She needed her mother, and her father was on duty. This must be when hands fold to pray, when they're otherwise of no use. Playing God is not a role I'm comfortable in, but Jody and I found ourselves choosing therapies that caused pain and might do more harm than good. You only get to know which in retrospect.

I was at J's side, reading to her, not from the Christian Scriptures but again from Junie B. Jones, stroking her head and scratching where she couldn't reach. Morphine made her itch. I supplied cold towels. She was coming to and breathing well. She was in pain. She wondered why there was a tube in her side, and began to favor that side physically.

We returned to Seven West, better late than never, a small reservoir in J's chest and a tube in her side. The initial doses of ATG and cyclosporine would wait another day to begin. She was hungry. She was cranky. Two clowns from the Big Apple Circus knocked on our door. They didn't ask to pray with us. One wore pants that squeaked. One wore pants that farted. I'd like to think there's a limit to the number of times a clown with farting pants can make me laugh, but I hadn't reached it yet.

In such a place, in such a time, the need for and the limits of religious faith become clearer. When an entire ward is asking for favors, does God roll his eyes? Is God ever cynical? What does he do with all those promises made during dark-night-of-the-soul moments such as J in pain trying to sleep while Tinky Winky sings "Turaluralura" on the other side of the curtain? Does God have a vig? Will a thick-necked Irish tough come to collect? I have faith that God won't break my knuckles or knees, because I may need them to pray. The prayer I have in mind is from the prophet John Prine: *Just give me one thing I can hold onto.*

CHAPTER THREE

The Hotel California

I can't tell Pac-Man from Ms. Pac-Man. Not anymore. Once, I knew both well. Table versions, first of Pac-Man, then of Ms. Pac-Man, were installed in a strip-mall bar in Tarzana, California, where in the early 1980s other sports writers and editors and I would drink assorted concoctions and play till last call or we ran out of quarters after putting out the next day's *L.A. Daily News* sports section.

Nearly a quarter-century later, Ms. Pac-Man and I became reacquainted in the Game Room of Seven West. The game was the same, except that it was free, and didn't end till a kid wanted it to. You wouldn't want to try that on a sports writer approaching last call.

J preferred singles, so mostly I'd watch her play. In the game, the player directs the Pac-Man through progressively challenging mazes, swallowing up white dots and the occasional bonus characters, ghosts who spend most of their time as Pac-Man's pursuer. By swallowing the four blinking energizers, Pac-Man becomes the pursuer and, for a few seconds, can swallow the ghosts and score major points. Wait too long, and the ghost becomes pursuer again and swallows Pac-Man. J got quite good at it, her score rising higher and higher.

The game was based on the human immune system, subconsciously if not intentionally: T cells working for you one minute, turning on you the next. We were playing for time, dashing through the maze in search of a blinking energizer. It felt good to have access to a game we could make continue as long as we wanted. Such power.

On Seven West, our hope rode in on, not an energizer, but a horse. Fevers had delayed treatment, but waiting longer became riskier. Anti-thymocyte globulin, derived from a horse, offered no cure, but might make J's condition survivable. There would be side effects. Doctors recommended that one nurse see Day 1 through, and a nurse who knew J well expected to be with her all day, watching closely for allergic reactions. That was the plan. But Pharmacy was slow getting the order together, and by the time the ATG arrived, General Pediatrics was at lunch and unable to test for allergic reaction. Heme-Onc came to the rescue. Jennifer Whangbo always rode to the rescue. She was like John Wayne in that way. Same initials, too. When all else failed, she was there. A welcome contrast to the swaggering, rounding intellectuals, hers was an attentive, soft-spoken brilliance, and her very presence brought comfort. She knew us like no other doctor caring for J.

The skin test showed no allergic reaction, and treatment began at 2:30 p.m. ATG is derived from horses or rabbits, and J was treated initially with the former, though in time we'd count on the rabbit's serum, if not its foot, to change our luck. After 30 minutes of the equine elixir, J got itchy, then hungry, craving white rice. I told the nurse I was leaving and ran across the street for steamed rice and a couple of packets of soy sauce. By the time I returned, J had the chills, lost her appetite and fell asleep. She started sweating and broke out in hives. The nurse slowed the flow of ATG, which inflicts side effects long before it does any good. What was intended to be a six-hour process took eleven. Platelets plummeted, if plummeting is possible from such a low starting point. This, too, was expected with ATG. J would get a bag of platelets each of the four days.

Since the surgery to insert the port and chest tube, she'd been protectively contorting her left side. The overnight nurses moved J to a less awkward position in bed, but this left her in pain, on continuous morphine, and she awoke in a damned if you do, damned if you don't state. Movement caused her pain, but she couldn't do things for herself. She needed help with everything but was wary of anyone poking about her. She gave me looks I interpreted as: *You're my dad, make them stop!* I hoped it would help when the chest tube came out later in the day. The fluid had drained from her lung. A seal had been achieved, a bullet dodged. J didn't look forward to the tube's removal, but knew she didn't have to leave bed for the procedure and would feel better when it was out. She still somehow trusted such assurances. I believe she just wanted there to be no more medical procedures of any kind for a while, a day even, but there wouldn't be a day like that any time soon.

A surgeon came to our room to remove the chest tube. Our roommate marched past to use the bathroom, leashed to an IV pole and followed by her dad. Craving privacy, J was agitated. There was tape to remove, sticky adhesive, stitches, and a tube the size of TV cable penetrating her side and going in maybe half a foot. J didn't want to get right to it. The surgeon was patient, and waited to receive her go-ahead. *Ow!* she said, and it was out.

GCSF is an acronym for granulocyte-colony stimulating factors. They're meant to boost white cell production, but they'd failed us and we discontinued GCSF. J wouldn't get jabbed in the leg for that drug, but that was the only positive.

The port had been in 72 hours, but a poorly functioning surgical IV remained in her foot. I don't recall the logic, only the uncomfortable fact. J hadn't been out of bed for days, and a morning walk inflamed the foot.

She winced getting into a wheelchair for an evening X-ray. She was weak and sore and bending to her left and keeping one arm tucked over the tube wound. Her body language put her age at about ninety.

A new roommate's mom was watching a reality cop show, and we drowned it out with "Charlie and the Great Glass Elevator" read by Eric Idle. J cracked up, laughing so hard she held her port side. Thank God her laughter was returning. She played with foam puzzle pieces, called Snafooz. Snafu stood for Situation Normal, All Fucked Up. I decided J didn't need to know this.

The last ATG infusion on October 3 brought fewer side effects, as doctors had predicted. At 5:50 p.m., just as the bell sounded to say the infusion was complete, Dr. Whangbo arrived with her welcome and calming smile. A physical therapist also stopped by to assess J. Groggy and grumpy, with a body bent like a comma, J did her best to cooperate. The therapist said she'd return the next day.

Jody posted: "*J tolerated her last day of ATG treatment yesterday very well: no fever, no chills, no hives. All around it was a great day. They took the IV in her foot out so she can walk around by herself. She had a bath. J just realized yesterday that she can't go to Pumpkinfest. It was upsetting. But I also know that Paul and myself are really good at creating a stimulating, creative, fulfilling environment for her right at Mom's place. We are so eager to be out of this hospital.*"

Through the window of Room 709, I had a view of Beth Israel Hospital's Shapiro Building, where in an OB/Gyn's office in 1997 I saw J's face for the first time, via ultrasound. I swear, she looked right at me.

Inside 709, J was lethargic all morning but perked up when the tutor arrived.

Doctors and nurses prepared us for outpatient visits to the CAT/CR, the Center for Ambulatory Treatment & Clinical Research at Children's, but we didn't hold our breath. CAT/CR is for outpatient care, and we showed no signs of becoming outpatients. J couldn't leave the hospital till the fever was gone, and though her fever would break, it wouldn't break for long.

In my erratic adaptation to this new normal, I was slowly learning to live more in the moment. Planning ahead fit poorly into that mindset. And yet we knew checkout day was coming, and when it did, we'd need to keep J away from more than moldy basements and snotty noses. The necessary environment: dry and dust-free. Avoid solvents, paint thinner, benzene, chemicals of any sort; avoid the zoo and playgrounds. The list of people, places and things wearing skull & crossbones was long and growing longer. During the first month out of the hospital, we were told, we couldn't go out at all, except to bring J several times a week to Children's Hospital, aka Infection Central, where we'd Purell often, have J wear a mask, zip through the lobby like a SWAT team and duck into a private room at CAT/CR ASAP.

The administrators on Seven West kept saying we should meet to prepare forms and get our marching orders, but Jody and I kept putting it off. Seven West had become our cocoon where we waited for our neutropenic butterfly to sprout white cells, and we weren't eager to emerge without some kind of immune defense.

J was eager to be well again. We talked about patience. I told her getting well from aplastic anemia would be a long process that would be frustrating, annoying and require lots of patience. I tried to choose my words carefully, as if I knew what the hell I was talking about. I didn't want this to be a lesson in do as I say, not as I do, and I was just as eager for her to be well again.

Jody posted: "*This afternoon, Paul was literally packing up our camp here to go home to Grandma Joan's when J spiked a fever. That means we'll be here at least through the weekend because she needs to be fever-free for 48 hours before we can go home. J was disappointed that we were not going home, but all of us agree it was better than going home and then turning right around and coming back through the Emergency Room.*"

My notes say J was afebrile all day on October 7. That is, she didn't have a fever. October 7 apparently was also the day I began using medical terms. I'd asked J's doctor what afebrile meant a day earlier. Now I knew. J's port got a good workout, taking in bags of red blood and platelets, recently harvested from the veins of people I'll never know. If they were yours, thanks.

J's neutrophils jumped from zero to seven, but I didn't get all febrile about it. Dr. Shannon said seven was the new zero. A body needs 500 neutrophils to hold its own against an infection. Zero to seven meant squat. Zero to 400, we could get little excited; 400 to a thousand, we could really start whooping it up, maybe shrug when somebody sneezed. Still, with zero to seven, there was movement, and where there's movement, there's hope. I didn't seek a second opinion on that.

Cousin Jessica and her husband John sent J a CD compilation. The Cars' "Shake It Up" was playing when Emily arrived.

I posted: "*J had a visit this morning from her cousin Emily. It was like throwing a switch on J's mood. After about 10 minutes, J told Emily "Stop making me laugh, you're making my port hurt." She was laughing when she said it. If only we can find a way to throw a switch on her bone marrow. Maybe the ATG/cyclosporine treatment will do the trick. That is our hope, but only time will tell. We've been making great use of a CD player brought to us by some First Parish friends. J just about knows the first Harry Potter by heart, and she's acquiring my appreciation for Eric Idle (reading Roald Dahl). We nearly did in the poor CD player by leaving it on a table under a humidifier. It dried out after a day in the window, and seems to have survived its marination. J let us watch some of the last Red Sox game, but lost her patience when Johnny Damon struck out with the bases loaded and we switched to "The Wild Thornberrys," which had a happier ending.*"

45

Among the chaplains, child-life specialists and assorted hope pur-veyors, Christina was an adept provider of compassion. A kind, sensitive and resourceful social worker, she had been in our room several times, developed a relationship with each of us and helped to ease our transition to Heme-Onc and the new normal. A woman of boundless empathy, Christina had a great sense of when it wasn't a good time, an important skill when it's your job to knock on doors where it's never a good time, only occasionally less bad. She said J was a candidate for Make-a-Wish. I thought Make-a-Wish focused on the hopeless, and I was desperately hopeful. Christina caught me right when I was inventing my blinders, and I lit into her. *J has a life-threatening illness, not a fatal illness,* I said in my *Don't let the screen door hit you on your way out* voice. Christina calmly, without offense, explained that Make-a-Wish had outgrown my limited and bleak view of its mission, and now reached out to kids with merely life-threatening illnesses. Since the funeral, I knew the difference.

So I reset my asshole circuit breaker and said we'd think about it. Jody and I discussed it, looked around Seven West at all the bald heads and bleak expressions, the families split in two, including a bereft woman with one son on Seven West and another child with a heart problem two floors up, who had to choose which one needed her more. We didn't have to choose. We considered the many blessings and resources within our own family, and declined Christina's offer. We could provide for J in ways some parents couldn't, and there were needier kids for Make-a-Wish to make something hopeful happen for.

In particular, one bald and diminutive resident of Seven West looked expectantly into the hallway every time I passed. He never had a parent visit, let alone spend the night, near as I could tell. Nurses were his family. He was like Fuzzy Stone from "The Cider House Rules." I wonder what came of Fuzzy.

Christina said she understood and dropped the subject. But she came back. Before making our decision, she said, we should consider what J was going through, and that Make-a-Wish's mission is to give such kids something to look forward to. I can't say for certain that her words were *something to look forward to,* but that phrase, that idea, stuck with me. I was trying to find my own way out of despair. Wallowing, it turns out, is an ineffective parental tool. Despair is nothing to see in the face of the parent for a kid trying to find a way to get better, who can't comprehend what's wrong in the first place, or why me? When you're going through repeated needle sticks and inspections and tests and watching substances red and yellow and clear drip from bags into a hole poked in your arm or wrist or foot or chest while prescribed starvation means all you get to swallow is some vile medicine whose clearest purpose is to make you writhe and wretch, and they still won't give you Tylenol because they want to see what the fever does. When teams of rounding doctors of various specialties daily trample your privacy at the very age it's beginning to matter.

We said yes to Make-a-Wish. J was in no hurry to decide what to ask for, but discussing possibilities gave us wings to ride on and, indeed, something to look forward to. We considered the usual suspects – DisneyWorld, or some other fun and cheerful place – and yet we'd done that already, and if I ever get over the horror of hearing Aaron Copeland emanating from ferns, maybe we'll do it again. J was fascinated with Mount Everest, and a trip there soon rose to the top of her list. But Everest rose above Make-a-Wish's comfort zone. Mine, too. A Disney Matterhorn is one thing, Everest quite another. J also had become fascinated with figure skating and the Olympics, with Irina Slutskaya in particular, so skating with Irina, or even just meeting her, became a consideration. I suggested front row tickets to Springsteen. Jody countered with Madonna. It became a running joke. Turns out, Make-a-Wish has good radar for parents horning in on a kid's wish.

Hanging prominently on our wall on Seven West was a poster of our neighbor's pond. Looking at the poster transported all three of back to our home, and reminded us of the hours J spent poking around in the water, looking for critters, learning to spot toad eggs and to leave them alone, finding garden snakes under rocks and salamanders under bark. A cardinal in our crab apple or a golden finch on a sunflower elicits a call from J to come quick and see. And so we thought about a wish with a future, one that assumed a return to health, during a time when nature was a fearful place. What could we do in our own yard to create a unique space for her to be in nature? Something that would give her that forward vision to see her way beyond the molds and spores and bacteria. Something without a Purell dispenser.

It became unnecessary for both of us to get a bad night's sleep, so Jody and I took turns leaving the hospital at night. I slept better than Jody amid the bells and beeps, and having left my newspaper job to be a stay-at-home dad, I seldom had an obligation to shape our schedule. So Jody's professional life, and the need to prepare for it, dictated who stayed. As J's comfort with the nurses and her environment grew, it mattered less to her which parent stayed. Though neither Jody nor I wished to be away for long, and we craved more time together, it was good to get out of the hospital environment for a few head-clearing hours, and perhaps enjoy a private conversation with a friend.

An IV inserted into J's port would last a few days before needing to be changed. She hated pokes and feared accessing the port would hurt, but Suzanne, a nurse fast rising to the status of Brooke, pulled it off without a tear. The trick was Emla, a white cream that numbed the skin and made a needle stick in the chest not such a big deal. *Did you bring the Emla?* would join *Did you Purell?* on our list of questions to always remember.

The port was no help with cyclosporine, a drug as crucial as it was befuddling. Cyclosporine had transformed organ transplantation, and we would count on it to keep the suspect T cells at bay indefinitely. It was dosed every 12 hours, and had to be taken on time because the level was checked at the 12-hour low. You want neither too much nor too little, but the correct dosage was elusive, as J burned through one dose rapidly, then barely put a dent in the next. Her levels charted like a San Andreas seismograph. The syrup smelled skunky and tasted vile. It was available as a caplet, but Heme-Onc insisted on the syrup, the "goop," till consistency was achieved. Sometimes J was a trooper and took it right down with a cranberry juice chaser. When it took too long, the time was duly noted on her chart, so the next draw and dose could be adjusted. Grapefruit juice does strange things to cyclosporine, so J's doctors banned it. No problem. J was about as eager for a glass of grapefruit juice as she was for skunky cyclosporine.

I posted from Children's Hospital: *"Jody says this is Fever City. I call it the Hotel California, where you can check out any time you like, but you can never leave. And though I'm beginning to believe the Radiology Department at Children's is a creation of Franz Kafka, I'm also in awe of the brain power here trying to sort out what's wreaking havoc on J, and moved by the care she's receiving from the nursing staff. J is doing her own IV/port flushes now, helped with a blood draw a short while ago, and holds her own with both nurses and doctors in conversation. The other day, as we answered a new doctor's questions, I couldn't remember the name of the medication she'd had an allergic reaction to a couple of weeks earlier, and went to look it up in my notebook. "It was the ambizome, Dad," said J, rolling her eyes. And, of course, it was. She may have gotten her rolling eyebrows from me, but not her ability to retain details. We're more or less moved in with Jody's Mom on Comm Ave. and feeling quite blessed to have such a place to go to while our renovation wraps up. Uncle Dave and Aunt Linda are on a mission to get our home ready for us. Dave has a specialist coming to make sure our heating/cooling ducts are free of dust or other potential problems, and rooms we once planned to carpet we're rethinking. Clearly, our sense of what is "clean enough" has changed for good. So long from our Longwood Avenue timeshare."*

Nurse Vicky did the impossible; she got an answer out of Radiology at 9 in the morning. Radiology postponed the MRI do-over a day, gave us a 12:30 p.m. appointment, and J didn't have to fast. Her chest and abdominal pain had eased, but her left shoulder was achy, so she wasn't in great spirits when her Grampa Gerry arrived. Still, they played games and had a visit, and I left to pick up a few things to take to Joan's and made calls about the warranty for our tub, which was newly installed and already leaking. I'd gotten a deal on a floor model. Bad call. Floor models are the generic drugs of plumbing fixtures.

Because of J's experience with nembutal, it was proposed that she try the next MRI without sedation. This apparently works with some kids, and she was game to try. Another bad idea. The MRI chamber looks like something Michael Jackson preserved himself in. It's essentially an open-ended coffin. The subject is strapped in tight and told not to move, and then the imaging begins and it gets scary. J made it into the chamber, but once the Nordic Death Metal music began, she started to quiver, and the MRI was stopped. I assumed we would calm her, sedate her with something other than nembutal, and try again. I was wrong. There was no one to administer anesthesia. We returned to Seven West, rescheduled and starved J yet another day. Don't get me started on Radiology.

Dr. Shimamura said she wanted to keep J off Tylenol because it masked fevers and complicated understanding of what was going on in her body. But this wasn't communicated to other docs. General Pediatrics ordered Tylenol whenever she spiked a fever. I headed it off. J awoke with abdominal pain and received codeine for it. Our infant roommate screamed sporadically through the night, though, and J was frustrated. So was I. J finally fell sleep around 5 a.m. with Eric Idle reading Willie Wonka in her headphones, then was awakened to take her cyclosporine. She was in no mood for it. I told her if she took it, I'd talk to the doctors about switching to pills. She squirted the cyclosporine into her mouth, swallowed—*Even goopier!*—gulped down some water, then tried to kill the taste with a mint chocolate. None of it stayed down long, so she had to take it all over. She had no fever, but her blood pressure was up.

Jody posted: "*Well, to make a long story short, the MRI became a CAT scan instead. The pictures showed an appendix that kinda sorta looks inflamed. They're wondering if it's appendicitis, but they don't know for sure. So they're just going to monitor her through the night and give her special medicines that combat the kind of bacteria in inflamed appendixes. They're taking a wait and see attitude. She has some of the symptoms of appendicitis but not all. Because her immune system is so fragile, they don't want to do surgery unless they're absolutely sure it needs to be done. She's resting very comfortably right now, which is great because last night was kinda rough. All quiet now in room 709. And for the first time in four weeks (yes we have been here 4 weeks), we have no roommate!! Amazing.*"

Away from the hospital, I called for a portable storage unit. Carpenters, electricians and heating people needed more room to maneuver in our garage.

I also researched eating disorders related to medical manipulations. J was NPO for the third day in four, and soon it would be four in five.

Lipids were nourishing her through the solution dripping into her new port, but J never mistook lipids for something to eat. Now she couldn't eat because doctors were concerned about her appendix and possible emergency surgery.

Had she enough platelets, they'd take no chances, schedule the minor surgery and remove the useless and troublesome organ. But she'd already shown how wrong surgery could go with her inability to clot. There was no minor surgery with J, so another antibiotic was assigned the task of making the inflammation go away. But as long as the potential for an appendix rupture and a dash to surgery existed, she couldn't eat. She got so giddy that she couldn't stop thinking about Pizza Stop and Burger King. We played cousin Jess's compilation CD; on "Everything Little Thing She Does Is Magic," Sting sang *ayo, ayo*. J smiled and told me, *It sounds like they're saying mayo. Mmm, mayo.* I know of no Police lyric that rhymes with lipid.

My notebook reads like a litany of symptoms and side effects. J was clear: *Don't put that on the Carepage!* Interspersed with the unmentionables were trends that seemed notable and worth remembering, drug names and dosing changes; a home renovation checklist.

I'd also written down a Carepage address of a kid down the hall who already had the challenge of Down syndrome and impending heart surgery when the leukemia reared up. When I first saw her, her lips and tongue were swollen and bleeding. She was my first view of that aspect of chemo. I don't recall her mom ever away from her side, though she made time to advise me, as we considered life outside the hospital, on nutritional ways to boost J's immune defense. I met many angels at Seven West. This mom was one. In time I would slip elderberry extract into J's fruit shake, and she'd go for oat bran a morning or two each week, but that bottle of aloe vera juice sat in Joan's fridge for ages. No way I could sneak that into a smoothie.

Hydralazine was added to J's daily cocktail. A nurse said it was a pneumonia preventative, but Wikipedia said it was for blood pressure. J also needed to swallow a thick yellow liquid known as atovaquone. It smelled like synthetic bananas and would be with us for quite some time. It went down easier than most. J's gums hurt when she ate, and we thought maybe it was a side effect of the cyclosporine, but at least she got to eat again: clear liquids first, then white solids. Crackers. Toast. *Mayo* ...

The docs pulled J off all antibiotics but zosin, for her appendix. Zosin seemed to be making surgery unnecessary. As of October 18, she'd been afebrile for four days. The cause never revealed, the fever was gone.

A chaplain dropped by unannounced. I wasn't sure what to do with him. Like the nun who came to pray with us before J's port surgery, it felt better to say OK and play along or pray along than to say go away. Maybe God hadn't forsaken us. But by all indications, no one on Seven West remembered to smear lamb's blood on their front door. On Seven West, the angel of mercy was at best passive aggressive.

The rooms on Seven West were wired for Internet, and we made good use. J and Emily connected regularly via Skype. Jody and I checked emails, posted Carepage updates and Googled drug names and therapies and began to understand getting your medical information from the Web is a bad idea.

J and I ordered a print online from the National Gallery of Scotland to give to Jody for Christmas. Two months earlier, while Jody participated in her psychology conference, J and I toured the National Gallery, where the permanent collection was full of Christian imagery and the Scots collection by comparison was notably shy of God, favoring landscapes and portraits of intellectuals. The 19th Century Scottish painter James Guthrie caught our eye with a rendering of the boardwalk at Oban, the ferry port to the Isle of Mull. The colors were muted, even dreary in comparison to other of his works, but the painting transported me back to a special place, and I hoped it would do the same for Jody. J concurred. I ordered a print.

J was prescribed magnesium, as cyclosporine was chewing hers up. Her ability to swallow pills continued paying off. Each new medicine came with its own side-effect warning, and it's hard for a kid to appreciate eventual benefits of drugs that make her feel lousy right away. But the cyclosporine achieved a certain consistency, so docs let her switch to pills. And although the first pill was big enough to choke a vacuum cleaner, cyclosporine also came in 25mg. J would sometimes need to swallow six or more twice daily, and the capsules had a skunkiness all their own, but they went down so much easier than the goop. J was proud that she'd learned to swallow pills; she knew from roommates and nurses on Seven West that it was a significant achievement. For Jody and I, this was a close second to the port-a-cath in making treatment tolerable. J's spirits were remarkably good now that she hadn't been NPO for a few days. She was eating well, and was unleashed from her IV pole.

I got the sense J was sick of being the patient. *How are you feeling?* She hated the question. She'd roll her eyes, then lay back and close them. She shut out the world. But it was the question that bothered her. If there was a procedure, accessing a vein or her port or giving a shot, she didn't want to be distracted. She didn't want the nurse to count to three; *Just do it.* She paid close attention but didn't want to be quizzed or monitored, and I monitored her constantly. I became aware of the need for me to take in everything but to do it in some faux nonchalant fashion, and to react strongly to nothing.

I needed to be like Jesus in that image with the eyes that open or close depending which angle you view him from. I needed my eyes to close from J's perspective. J was developing a need for privacy, and it was violated multiple times daily.

Jody helped her understand the necessity of all that was being done to her, and to see the positive aspect and potential of it; her illness shouldn't happen to anyone, but it did, and lucky for us to have been so near such remarkable understanding and care.

And yet J had ample cause for anger, so we let her be pissed off when necessary. A new verb: NPO'd.

Jody posted: *"Last night, J and I watched a wonderful DVD that her classmates at Lincoln School made. Wow! J got a kick out of the funny anecdotes that the kids told and I got teary-eyed just seeing footage of her classroom again. It was TREMENDOUS hearing about all that the kids have been doing. J was happy to see that she's been keeping up on reading the same books that her classmates are reading. And she was quite intrigued about the bat they saw on a field trip. In a bit, we will finish viewing the movie "Harry Potter and the Sorcerer's Stone." We started it last night and J really liked it (she knows the whole story by heart from the audio book CD), until Harry arrived at his Griffindor room at Hogwarts. It started to feel too scary, so we decided to turn it off and watch the rest in the light of day."*

It was difficult to tell friends and family to stay away, or to give them the third degree about symptoms and contacts should they come to visit. I trust people to do the right thing, but my daughter's well-being had never been so precarious. So I got used to making certain no one in her presence would put her at risk. I even reminded doctors to use Purell. J never had any reluctance. She learned to look out for herself.

But what if the risk was me? In the fall, when the cool, dry wind blows through New England and mold is in the air amid the swirling and fluttering leaves, I fairly regularly sniffle and sneeze and rub my eyes and blow my nose. Before J was so sick, it was easy to assume the symptoms were due to allergy, not a virus or worse. I began to take my own temperature every day as a precaution, and I washed and Purell'd obsessively.

I called my own doctor. There were shortages of flu shots, and I wanted to be sure I got mine. My doctor was in a large practice, one that could seem more committed to insurance efficiencies than to patients. I was told they did not offer flu shots. The best they could do was direct me to a website with a link to clinics that did offer them. I found a pharmacy on the first floor of my doctor's building. I told the pharmacist that my doctor's staff was unaware of the clinic, and perhaps they should let the doctors in the building know. The pharmacist was taken aback; he already had faxed the practice twice.

I like my doctor. He's considerate, smart and takes the time to listen. But he does seem to be part of a bureaucracy in which the best interests of the patient get lost. This is important, as a patient, to know. A patient needs some awareness of the ways a system compromises a doctor. It was a lesson I'd get again, in a decision with greater ramifications, within months.

J posted: "*Hi Friends. It's J (with Jody typing). Today was one of the greatest days in the hospital. One of my favorite nurses Brooke is my nurse tonight. And my dad brought my red pants and my red shirt so I really look like a devil with my devil horns and spear. So you can see today has been a really great day. My grandma Lucy and grandpa Gerry came over and we baked mini apple pies. They were really good. We finished them all in one night. We got to use the oven in the hospital that only the nurses get to use so my grandparents didn't have to go back to the house to bake them. I'm doing fine, how about you? Love, J"*

When rounding doctors gathered around J and discussed her situation, she'd check my reaction. I became aware of the influence I had over the way she heard and processed information about her own health. Through a series of emotional breakdowns, beginning with my exit from the emergency room when J's nostrils were being cauterized, I came to see myself as serving no useful purpose to my daughter, who desperately needed me to serve a useful purpose. I wondered what it would feel like to a child to be surrounded by doctors asking questions of the life and death sort and to look up and see only fear in the face of your father. I'm not sure I can truly comprehend that feeling, but I know it feels like defeat. My daughter's body was deteriorating, and I was feeling sorry for myself. She needed me, and I was self-absorbed. I knew I was at the mercy of the nurses and doctors to save J's life, but she was looking to me for clues, for ways of handling this information, and if it was overwhelming for a 50-year-old man, how was his seven-year-old daughter expected to handle it? I needed to do something about my own ability to process and comprehend the flood of information about the chaos inside J's body. Educated decisions would need to be made, and soon. So I parked my emotions. I don't know where I put them, I just packed them away, like some ancient file on a floppy disc.

The night following J's twin surgeries, while Jody slept with J, the images of her agony were working themselves to the surface as I prepared for bed. I had no wish to revisit the day's events; I wished only to escape them and return fresh to J's side in the morning. Tucked away on a sofa bed in the Seven West family room, the small room in which Drs. Shimamura and Whangbo had given J's illness a name and revealed a plan, I watched a Dylan documentary by Martin Scorsese. *Your old road is rapidly agin'.*

Still wired when the documentary ended, I found the novel "Knots & Crosses" on a shelf. I'd been wanting to discover Ian Rankin since Edinburgh. I read until my eyes closed and my mind shut off. *Please get out of the new one if you can't lend your hand.* Dylan and Detective Rebus kept the day's images at bay until I passed out. I'd call on them again.

Father of one, I'd never heard a biological clock ticking, but I began to feel a pounding. Waiting and hoping for J's numbers to climb and show us that we were part of the 70 percent success of the immunosuppressants, I couldn't stop thinking about what if it didn't work. It wasn't a cure. Only transplant offered cure. There was an international system in place to link us with possible donors of bone marrow, and yet literature said having a matched sibling was better. And what if no stranger matched with J? If the immunosuppressants failed, it would be at least a couple of months before we'd know, and bone marrow transplant works best when performed within a year of diagnosis, and after as few transfusions as possible. And so, if we were to have a second child, there was no time to waste. I freaked Jody out with my manic urgency. I desperately needed an answer to a question set in stone on a tablet of moral ambiguity.

Jody and I asked Akiko Shimamura for a meeting, and she made time for us quickly. In a small borrowed office, I told her my concern about wasting time and my need to better understand whether creating a new life was in J's best interest, our best interest – in the *new being*'s best interest.

Patiently, calmly, Akiko explained our situation, as she saw it. In creating a new child though normal means, there would be a one in four chance of that sibling being a suitable donor for J. However, in a lab, scientists can take a fertilized egg and manipulate it at the right time in the splitting process, and greatly improve chances of a match. That miracle of science was the simple part. The tricky part was in the ethics of such a creation; not the scientific ethics, but the personal, parental ethics. What if we managed to create a match with a Down gene or some other genetic problem discovered under a microscope? Then what? And yet the bottom line transcended all concerns – I wanted to save J's life, and if there were a way to do that with a reasonable chance of success, I wanted to do it.

Thank God we had Akiko to turn to. The conversation had Jody in tears and me in knots, and yet we both left satisfied that saving J did not require that we create another child. Akiko said they'd already done a check of the donor registry, and J had many potential matches. Hundreds. The donor registry is quite the bigot. It counts on volunteers and favors white-skinned people with minimal twists and turns in the DNA. Both Jody and I are of Northern European ancestry. Further, Akiko said, the ability of doctors to control engraftment had improved so greatly that a well-matched, unrelated donor held nearly as much hope as a sibling for J. This is not what some sources on the Web said, but we trusted Akiko.

Peter and a pregnant Rachel, Jody's sister, came to visit. J always lights up around them, and the idea that she'd have a new cousin within days added to her excitement. Cousins are especially great when you don't have a sibling. We discussed the concept of saving the cord blood. Peter and Rachel were way ahead of us.

I posted: *"We think we have good news but know better than to jinx ourselves. As J told the hematologists Drs. Bennett and Vrooman this morning, "Don't use the D-word or you'll give me a fever." Still, we anticipate this is our last night at Children's. Our friend Dr. Michael Shannon stopped by to say hi, and we shared our news about our impending parole. He was happy for us, but even happier when J showed him how to play Pac-Man. She'll miss that game almost as much as the nurses on Seven West. Michael's visit is just one example of how great the doctors are at Children's. Here's another: Last Friday, Sanjiv (Call me Sonny) Harpavat dropped in for the last time as her daily pediatric contact. He's got two months to go before he can call himself a doctor, but he's already gifted with kids. He spent the better part of an hour doing origami with J. Sometimes she gets tired of all the doctors and all their questions and pokes and prods and pills, but when they sit down and do origami, all is forgiven."*

The D-word is discharge. Use of it became a joke – another He Who Must Not Be Named. The word surgery also held that role with J, but the S-word was no joke. The very thought of surgery frightened her, and with good reason. Our avoidance of saying discharge was based not on fear, but on frustration, and maybe denial, as more than once we'd prepared to leave only for a fever to return and delay our parole. With J in a wheelchair and mask, ready to venture into the world outside, a large cart stacked with all our stuff, we made it to the button on the Seven West wall; with one push, the doors would swing open on our corridor to freedom. J said she felt hot. Brooke shot me the eyebrows and got a thermometer. We turned around.

But on October 25, the fever never came. I began taking things off the walls. I took down the poster of J's beloved pond, rolled it up and slid it into a protective sleeve. I took down the origami cranes from J's friends. I took down the stuffed animals from the IV pole, where J had created hammocks using hospital masks. I took down the photos and cards. I packed up, filled out forms, went over instructions related to J's home care, and then waited for the inevitable, but the inevitable gave us the day off. We pushed the button, the Seven West doors swung open, and in a half hour we were inside Grandma Joan's apartment. No fever, and all I could think was, be careful what you ask for.

Seven West was a pay-it-forward kind of place, where empathy and kindness were the only infectious things not kept in isolation and where the humility, compassion and clarity of purpose took my breath away. We had left, and were now on our own. Joan and J and Jody were excited. I was nervous. No one named Brooke or Suzanne or Jenn was at our beck and call. Dr. Whangbo wouldn't poke her head in and see how we were doing.

Joan had scotch. I love my mother-in-law.

I posted: *"We're home. We're glad. We're pooped. More tomorrow."*

CHAPTER FOUR

Now What

Through the east-facing window in J's new temporary bedroom, in the rear of her grandmother's artful and art-filled Back Bay apartment, we could see over the rooftops of neighbors to the Golden Dome, under which the politics of Massachusetts are conducted. The dome glistened on sunny winter days. From the west-facing window in Jody's and my new temporary bedroom, we could see the Prudential Building, lighting up depending on the mood and season to say GO SOX! or GO PATS! or for a few philanthropic nights during the holidays, MAKE-A-WISH! I closed my eyes and wished: GO NEUTRO-PHILS!

Also from our window, down the Commonwealth Mall and into the horizon, we could see the Citgo sign near Fenway Park, magnificent, near-blinding sunsets, and westerly storms bearing down. The north window in Joan's art studio revealed more apartments, some with manicured rooftop gardens but mostly blocking a view of the Charles River.

To the south, the light atop the Hancock Building would tell us what was headed our way. With a growing metaphorical interest in predicting changes in the weather, we googled the poem decoding the Hancock's weather report, printed it and taped it in the window beside Joan's piano: *Steady blue, clear view. Flashing blue, clouds are due. Steady red, rain ahead. Flashing red, snow instead.* Come Spring, flashing red could also mean the Sox had been rained out, but we wouldn't be in Joan's apartment long enough to shift from snow to Sox. By baseball season, we'd be enamored of all things Seattle, followers of the Mariners still licking our wounds from how the refs screwed the Seahawks in the Super Bowl.

Joan has a passion and a keen eye for art, and has infused her apartment with compelling and fanciful images and figures. There's Lydia, a life-size figure in carved wood of a woman seated and holding a bird. Lydia has startled many a guest, and has become family. A bronze crocodile greets visitors, and provides a place to sit and take off boots, beneath a blue basset hound's mournful stare. Paintings by three friends add up to a triptych capturing the stunning panorama of Joan's oceanside summer home in Martha's Vineyard. Wanting to brighten J's bedroom, Joan found a Vineyard artist to create a mobile of perhaps a hundred butterflies.

Classical is her music of choice, the earlier the better, but Joan joined me one night to watch an early-70s Springsteen performance on WGBH. It failed to clarify for her my passion for the artist, but she gave me a reissued "Born to Run" for my birthday, and I played it when she wasn't around. *Oh come take my hand. We're riding out tonight to case the promised land.* Joan arranged her studio for J to make art for hours, complete with Grandma's insightful guidance and with the occasional friend cleared to share air space.

About the only thing our new home didn't feature was a bedside button to push and immediately bring Brooke or Susanne or Jenn to us. Children's Hospital was a mile and light years away. On Seven West, J's environment was clean and safe. The room was mopped down daily, sheets changed, bathroom scrubbed, meds monitored, IV lines flushed and disinfected. That sanitized hospital smell is aromatherapy for the immunologically lacking.

J paid such close attention to all details, especially as related to meds and blood products infused through her port, and became expert at Heparin flushes. Not so her parents. Jody and I had watched the procedures with regularity, but paying attention and the actual doing are such separate acts. When the device in your hand connects to your daughter's blood system, knowledge and competence are lost with regularity and suddenness along the long and winding road from your brain to your hands. The Seven West nurses endeavored to train us—*Oops!* and we'd all have a nervous chuckle, except maybe J—but the training always was under that nurse's watchful eye. We had backup. To find myself now, in Joan's apartment, without my Brooke Button, shaking and trying to look calm and connecting J to an antibiotic doser, struggling to recall the code the visiting nurse instructed me to punch in to keep an alarm from going off, caused mood swings I'd like not to experience again. Jody would second that. J, too.

A week before Halloween, I snuck away to church for the first meeting of the committee on ministry. First Parish was a good place to take my mood swings. Reverends Jim and Martha were just beginning their shared ministry, and I'd spent countless hours over two years on the search committee that brought them to Brookline. I hadn't anticipated testing their pastoral skills quite so soon.

Unitarianism tends to be defined, by the more mainstream and traditionally religious, by the dogma and beliefs rejected by members when they left some other religion, and certainly my beliefs are shaped as much by the aspects of Catholicism I've abandoned as what I've come to embrace. Mom used to say that whenever two or more people gathered in Jesus' name, he was present. I don't question the truth of that for her, but it's not my truth. And yet that belief lives in my own sense of divinity, found in the spiritual connection between humans. Maybe it's a distinction without a real difference. Unitarianism's focus on the interconnected web of all existence resonates with that. Jody and I are soul mates, *anam cara*, connected in a profound and even divine way that I appreciate increasingly over time. This sense, this belief, gave me confidence our relationship would survive our ordeal. J and I share a spiritual connection that is no less profound. Heaven on earth, I'd call it.

Mom had this other saying—*Offer it up*. It meant that in time of pain or hardship, when trouble seemed too much to bear, I could simply hand the burden over to God. *Let go, and let God*, in other words. Mom gave so much power to statues and relics, scapulars and crucifixes. The God she told me of and so fervently believed in herself, the one waiting by the phone like some supernatural 911, no longer existed for me. And yet from early in J's illness, I felt comfort and support from a source that never revealed itself, and it was sustaining. It didn't help me make sense of what was occurring, but it helped in my acceptance and engagement. It was foundational.

"A mother and young daughter were residents of Seven West when we arrived and when we left: The daughter sitting up in her hospital bed, head bald from the chemo, lips puffy, bloody and oozy, her mother beside her, looking up and smiling as J and I and the IV pole walk by. The mom said she'd pray for us, add us to her list. I've done enough rejecting in my adult life that I didn't want false comfort for myself or for J, but I did want comfort, solace, support, hope. And if somebody I like believes it and doesn't get heavy-handed or overly righteous about it, I don't question where the plea is directed. Not even the doctors could say they'd make everything OK. They promised to do all that they could, but they could do no more. So the mom said she'd pray for us, and I said thanks. Where else are you going to go?"

In setting priorities for its new ministers, Brookline's small but vibrant congregation hoped to see growth and yet somehow maintain the intimacy and connectedness. The committee on ministry became a place where the ministers could speak in confidence, share perceptions, explore and teach about living in right relations (Unitarian for honest and straightforward) and what it meant to be in community, to ask questions and begin learning what our evolving congregation really wanted to be. Because of J's illness, I'd miss most of the first year, both of the committee work and the new ministry. Perhaps that was for the best, as I had a new conception of what it meant to be in community. From an immune-suppressed perspective, it meant being at risk. The interconnected web had become a bacterial swamp. Safety was in isolation.

J asked about her treatment and the prospects of getting back to normal. My reply satisfied neither of us. J's 'crit was 31.5 several days after a red blood transfusion, which was encouraging, until Dr. Whangbo said it probably meant she wasn't drinking enough fluids. Dehydration causes false readings.

Dr. Shimamura said no taxis, but yes to trick or treating, so long as the conditions were right: warm, dry and no wind; no entering houses. J would go trick-or-treating with cousin Emily. Her friend Ellie wanted to join them. J and Ellie had been trick-or-treating together for half their lives, but Dr. Shimamura said no. *The one-kid rule.* Ellie's parents were trustworthy and responsible, Ellie herself was healthy, and saying no felt lousy. But our margin of error was gone. J got to go out in her devil costume and watch other kids parade by with fake blood pouring from fake head wounds. J made it as far as her grandparents' house as a devil, but it was getting cold, and soon she was a devil in a blue parka. Halloween in a parka wasn't what she had in mind, and she let me know. But this Halloween, I went as a hard ass. We passed cousin Michela, Emily's sister, out with several friends; the small crowd freaked me out, and I kept J moving. There's a polite way to do that; I hadn't found it yet.

Jody caught a cold. This meant J's mother had become the kind of person she couldn't be around. We talked it over and decided Jody didn't have to move out; distance, hand washing and Purell would suffice.

Jody might as well have had leprosy, the distance we maintained.

I posted: *"One of the hard things about J's condition is that it means she needs to live in a cleaner environment, which doesn't necessarily mean I have to be better about picking up my socks and not letting the dishes stack up in the sink (although both have been suggested), but it does mean she can't live with animals for a while, and perhaps for even longer than a while. So her buddy Abigail and her family stepped forward to offer a home to Heart & Flower, J's beloved guinea pigs. As for our cat Carlin Favre, he's done nicely up until now living amid the renovation, being fed by Uncle Dave, and sponging off neighbors. But then this week two things happened. One, Carlin followed Uncle Dave home. And Two, it snowed. Clearly, Carlin needed a more reliable home. And we've found one—again, right on our own street. Neighbor Peggy, our garden guru and someone who has known J since she was an infant, has adopted Carlin for as long as we need. Given Carlin's nature of going door to door and walking in whenever one opens, living three doors down from us will be much like living at our home. Despite all the upheaval in his life, Carlin remains a contented cat. And a VERY well fed one."*

For the exterior of our house, Jody wanted apricot with eggplant trim. I said she wasn't choosing shoe colors. I wanted a quarter-to-midnight blue with platinum trim, a combination the architect proposed and which I loved. J was the tiebreaker. She backed me up. Jody got apricot and eggplant in her office and the basement. Rooms with a shoe.

J's new cousin Myles was born as November 2 became November 3. We'd had an easy day at the CAT/CR, which produced the welcome news that J had recovered the weight she'd lost during her hospitalization and that she needed neither platelets nor red cells—in fact, the attending said it was time to lower her threshold for transfusions, and let her descend deeper into the danger zone before intervening. So J and I wandered across Longwood Avenue from Children's to Beth Israel to meet the half-day old Myles, born in the same hospital where J came into the world. To visit Myles and his parents, J wore a mask the whole time, through the lobby, onto the elevator, and I'm not sure which of us was more nervous in the uncontrolled environment, but J got to hold her new cousin maybe a dozen hours into his life. His parents saved the cord blood, more with a sense of its potential than for any particular need. Wish I'd thought of that.

Aunt Wrapping Paper sent us a Peanuts-themed Monopoly game. J chose Woodstock as her game piece. I went with Snoopy. We assigned Jody Lucy at the 5 cent psychiatry booth. J's emerging piano talent made her more Schroeder than Woodstock, and I'm Linus in ways I don't want to think about. But Jody will forever be Lucy at the psychiatry booth.

Though an ornery neighbor one floor up would disagree, Joan has a marvelous piano in her apartment, situated in a bright, sunny spot, and one of the few aspects of J's pre-aplastic anemia life not interrupted for long were lessons with Julie. Prior to her illness, J had made remarkable progress, and Julie was clear in telling us of her talent and the value in creating good practice habits. J had balked at the daily practice, and yet she also reveled in her rapidly emerging talent.

Julie's comprehension and meticulous respect for J's vulnerability put all three of us at ease with the idea that Julie would come to us to continue the lessons. She made that effort not only because she saw potential in J but because she cared deeply and wanted to help make the isolation less isolating. And so once or twice a week, Julie would come to Joan's apartment and teach.

Lessons were cancelled with regularity, either by me for a return to CAT/CR or by Julie because there's not enough Purell in the world to protect a piano teacher from multiple kids daily sharing her keyboard. At the slightest sign of symptoms, Julie would call and explain and reschedule. We got used to cancellations.

Lena, a tutor from the classroom J should have been in, also was conscientious and would call with the sniffles. Same with Peggy, a yoga instructor found by Lucy to help get J some physical activity. These were more contacts than J's doctors recommended, and Jody and I struggled with who and how many were acceptable. We never found a consensus; Jody's comfort pretty much guaranteed my discomfort, and vice versa. The simplest, clearest rule from doctors allowed nobody inside the house who wasn't immediate family. And yet we knew neutropenic kids from big families with multiple siblings coming home from school daily carrying who knows what. Jody and I decided to define immediate family on the liberal side, to consider J's emotional health along with her physical health, and we agreed that if either of us had misgivings, we'd cancel. We were dreadfully inconsistent, but consistency is the hobgoblin of little minds. Emerson, a Unitarian with a healthy immune system, said that.

To start their lessons, Julie often would play a piece to give J an idea of how it ought to sound and how attending to fundamentals and learning to read notes could develop a sound that transcended the mechanics. Julie's rapid runs on the keyboard were too fast for Joan, who told me this with a look I associate with fingernails on a chalkboard. In response, I told her a Jack Nicklaus story. Many years removed from sportswriting, and after years in arts journalism, I still know more about sports than culture. And I remember Jack Nicklaus describing teaching kids the game of golf. He didn't care how they gripped the club, He didn't care how they swung the club. He didn't care whether their body was in alignment with the target. Eventually he would care, but not until they'd learned to love the game. I told Joan I thought J was learning to love the piano. But Joan doesn't know golf, and Bach never said *Grip it and rip it.* I might as well have been speaking Farsi.

Joan had an obvious affection for Julie, though, and the tact and talent to express a difference of opinion without becoming disagreeable. She made her point. Julie and J got on with the lesson.

Jody posted: "*J was admitted to Children's Hospital last night with a fever. It was 101 F, which is the cutoff for taking her in. (I think Paul and I took her temperature 5 times!) She needs to be in the hospital because she doesn't have enough disease-fighting white blood cells to fight off whatever it is that is causing the fever. They will do lots of tests on her blood to figure out what it is and, in the meantime, give her broad-based antibiotics. We've been here before!*"

The route to Children's Hospital from the home in Brookline to which we hoped soon to return begins with a short walk to Walnut Street, then east a couple of blocks to the Philbrick House. The current residents of the Philbrick House own a farm and run a mail-order business sending bulbs and seeds to green thumbs in leafy neighborhoods who know the potential of such things. The former residents for whom the house is named gave the place its historic significance as a stop on the Underground Railroad. You plant your seed, you see what grows.

In educating myself for the ministerial search, I became aware of the Philbricks as more than a name on a plaque on Walnut Street. For me, their role at my church is frozen in an incident in the 1800s. Typical of the time, white families owned pews at First Parish and there was a section in the rear reserved for blacks. The white Philbricks wanted a black woman to sit in their pew. Other members of the church didn't like it and said so. The minister, caught in the middle, sided with the majority pew owners, those pious white faces settled into the hard dark wood, praying before a cross and ignoring their own persecutions. Rather than go along with that, Philbrick left the church. Beyond respect for that visionary integrity, I suspect this story has stuck with me for the notion that one might deem a church wrongheaded and opt out. Sounds simple enough.

Past the Philbrick House, it's a couple blocks more to Jody's sister's house, home to J's surrogate-sibling cousins, then past the God Is Love apartment church, on past the Dunkin Donuts and the old Firehouse on Route 9 with its Never Forget 9-11 banner, under the closed and drippy pedestrian bridge and past the subsidized apartments and the high-rise Brook House, then left onto Brookline Avenue, which takes you as far as Fenway Park, Boston's shrine to hope and faith, but to get to Children's Hospital you stop well short of the Red Sox stadium. Turn right on Longwood Avenue and in two blocks you're there.

It's a twenty-minute walk. Driving can take that long, too, depending on time of day. Sometimes when we'd drive, we'd get stuck at a light on Brookline Avenue, come to a stop alongside a city limits sign, and J would point out that I was in Boston and she was in Brookline. Then the light would change, and we'd be in the same place again.

One Sunday morning, I took the walk in reverse, from Children's to First Parish, and along the way, somewhere near the city limits sign, I passed a park where two teenagers I recognized were out with their dogs. One was a young woman whose parents I remembered from our early days at the church. We'd watched the parents light candles and update the community on their daughter's cancer treatment. The young woman, perhaps four at the time, had been in Children's, on the same floor and perhaps in the same room where J was now. She was treated for what had been an incurable cancer, but the Children's/Dana-Farber doctors were altering the nature of the incurable. Treatment was long, harsh, and successful. A decade later I walked past this young woman out with her dog and a friend on a Sunday morning. I smiled, took a deep breath, and my lungs filled with a hope grounded in faith and science.

I love that walk. I take it sometimes now, to go to the donor center to give platelets to assist some godforsaken unknown, though not every two weeks, which is how often I'm eligible to stop someone's bleeding. I should be there every two weeks.

I walked when J was admitted. Outpatient, we drove. Sometimes I'd use the valet service at Children's, but that meant waiting in the cold in a crowd once the appointment was over, since the crowded lobby was not an option and gridlock was a regular event. And so at first we parked in the structure across Longwood Avenue from Children's, climbing up and up and up, unless the parking god smiled on us and we scored a spot on a lower floor. Walking out of the parking structure onto Longwood would be our first blast of humanity, and I'd check that J's mask was securely in place, and try not to seem paranoid about it.

Such is the traffic in cars and anxiety that the entrance to Children's is one of the rare intersections in Boston where pedestrians wait for the walk signal. But waiting at a light in a crowd of uncertain wellness is not on any list of acceptable behavior for the immune suppressed and those who love them, and few places posed a greater risk of exposing my mask of reassuring calm. More often we'd take our chances and pull our car into queue for the drop-off circle, wait our turn amid the fumes, then hand the keys over to a valet, don the mask, and dash through the revolving door and into the large and bustling lobby of Children's Hospital, with its Au

Bon Pain and CVS and gift shop and fast-walking lab coats and crowded waiting areas and wailing babies and goopy-nose toddlers and frantic or demoralized parents in line at the parking kiosk.

We'd hear someone hacking loudly or sneezing in our general direction, and we'd give each other a look complete with rolled eyebrows and walk a little faster up the stairs to the elevator, also invariably crowded, so we'd take the stairs up the three flights, except on those days when J needed red blood and her energy was sagging. Then we'd take the elevator, crowd be damned.

Upon arrival at the CAT/CR, our first stop was at the Purell dispenser. Then we'd check in with Shannon, who took little notice of me, so intent was she on greeting "Angel Eyes," as she called J. Among the staff at Children's, there's this one personality type who gets it that it's the kid who needs the understanding, empathy and attention, and parents will just have to understand. Shannon was this type of person. She was a teacher, consciously or otherwise helping a frazzled and frantic parent redirect focus to where it belonged. After we'd run a gantlet of infectious risk to get to the CAT/CR, Shannon would welcome J with a larger than life smile, J would smile back through her mask, through her angel eyes, and we'd both exhale and head off to a private room. I'll probably never see Shannon again. I'll never forget her.

Between November 2005 and mid-March 2006, trips to CAT/CR were frequent. The appointments could begin slowly, if some other patient had priority needs, or if I'd forgotten to apply the Emla before leaving home. Emla cream needs a half-hour or 45 minutes to take effect. I didn't forget often, but when I did there were consequences, with J paying them, like that time a late-night fever returned us to Children's Emergency and, because it was a busy night in the ER and they didn't get to us immediately and when they did the nurse was no candidate for Seven West when it came to accessing a port or any other quality in putting a child and parent at ease and the Emla wore off and I didn't insist on applying more and waiting and the access went badly and J cried and I swallowed another moment I'll get around to forgiving myself for eventually.

But even the best nurse has bad days. One of J's favorites poked twice into the port without successful draw. This made no sense, as the port was a big target and seldom unforthcoming. But the IV needle seemed to be bouncing off the surface like bullets off Superman's chest. J was scared and couldn't hide it. The nurse was apologetic, and at a loss for what was going wrong. She'd done this with J so many times without a hitch. Today, two hitches. She had her supervisor take the third poke. Blood flowed.

At Fenway Park, 1 for 3 is a good day. At CAT/CR, not so much.

Nice word, access; simply descriptive yet euphemistic. They put access in the title of cable channels you have to pay extra for. When I was a sports writer, access meant I could get near certain people whose fame necessitated a shield from the general public. Access meant I could stand in the locker room after a game and ask questions of Kareem Abdul-Jabbar or Julius Erving, sit in a courtside seat as Magic Johnson and the Lakers took down the 76ers in the NBA finals, and if I was lucky on a road trip, access got me bumped to first class. Access meant playing golf with Bill Sharman one day and Johnny Mathis another, having a Molson with a young Wayne Gretzky and a few of his mates, interviewing Jack Nicklaus and then getting him to sign a book about his last Masters victory for Dad's birthday.

Access meant playing golf at Augusta National the morning after Larry Mize chipped in to beat Greg Norman. Back then, the way those athletes performed under pressure seemed so impressive, so courageous. Later, access meant getting John Hiatt on the phone to talk about his music and saying thanks for writing "Have a Little Faith" and telling him it was Jody and my first dance at our wedding reception. Access was a pass to Aerosmith's small-club gig. This access required no cream to deaden pain. As Jody transitioned from student to bread winner, I gave that access up for more access to my family. I became a stay-at-home dad.

Access came to mean something inflicted on my daughter on a regular basis—accessing her blood system, to take or to give, to assess or infuse. I liked access better as a noun. J was accessed to test her cyclosporine level, to restore her blood or platelets with a transfusion, to check what was there or wasn't, and why. In the early days of her illness, before the port, access was unpleasant at best. The port-a-cath changed that, made the process tolerable, and yet every time a nurse performed the procedure, I marveled at J's nonchalance. She'd be asked if she preferred to look away, if she'd like to watch TV or something to wrestle her conscious mind away from the fact that someone was about to thrust a needle into her chest. *Would you like me to count to three?* But J didn't want the count, the TV, the distraction; she wanted to observe. *Just do it.* J said that more times than I can recall.

I watched it so many times, I became Emla'd to the process, but every once in a while, I'd watch and shudder as the nurse, gloves on, prodded the skin over the port with her left index finger, trying to find just the right spot, then penetrated so near to the heart with a needle held between her right thumb and index finger, then screwed a tube onto the connector emerging from her chest and drew the first few cc's of what J had so goddam little of. Near as I could tell, the whole process tended not to be eventful for J, and once accessed, she'd ask me for Sudoku from the day's Boston Globe, or maybe to watch some TV, or for the Roll-up Piano her Aunt Wrapping Paper had sent her in one of those large boxes with who knows how many other individually wrapped packages inside, so she could work on *Ode to Joy*.

They say the marvel of a port-a-cath is that it can be penetrated a thousand or so times before it needs to be replaced. That's a lot of needle penetrations under a child's nose.

I posted: *"ANC stands for "absolute neutrophil count." Neutrophils are a white blood cell with a particular infection-fighting specialty, and you've probably got 40,000 or so of the little guys. For most of the past two months, J has had more fingers on her right hand that she's had neutrophils. Among the parents and friends at Seven West, it's an oft-heard question: "How are your counts?" Most of the time, a roll of the eyes is all the answer you receive. You try not to get too caught up in the frequent CBCs because the numbers tend to be either painfully and consistently low or something of a roller coaster. But it's hard not to refuel hope where you can, and J's neutrophils have been performing a bit lately. Today the count was 290, more than double what it was less than a week ago. Her periods between transfusions of red blood cells and platelets are getting a bit longer. Despite the prolonged periods without food while in the hospital, she weighs more than she did when this ordeal began. All of which is to say, we're feeling pretty optimistic today, and felt you ought to know."*

In CAT/CR, once the initial blood draw was made, the IV stayed in place, and we would settle in and wait to hear the results, which would determine whether we would stay only an hour or so, be deaccessed, and leave; or stay another hour or two for platelets, four for red cells or into the evening for a daily double.

Platelets had no noticeable effect on J, though the safety they brought buoyed both of us. Red cells were unmistakable. When she was running low on red cells, J was hard to get out of bed, hard to get moving and motivated to do little but stare at the TV. Once she'd received the red cells, even during the transfusion, she was bouncing off walls, and if she had the TV on, it was background noise for some creative endeavor. The problem with those days was that she'd be all ramped up just as we were leaving the CAT/CR, and though we'd been sitting around for hours, I was in no state to engage her enthusiasm. J developed the means for staying active and creative even when there was no one to play with. She always preferred having another human—cousin, friend, parent or grandparent—to interact with, but if I was only one available and had my head buried in the *New York Times* or an Ian Rankin novel or some other alternate universe, she entertained herself.

Along came Thanksgiving. Out of the hospital and relatively stable, gratitude came easy. I posted:

For neutrophils.

For doctors and nurses who get you by without them.

For intellectual brilliance and simple empathy.

For science.

For faith.

For wise counsel.

For hospital policy that lets parents stay with an ill child (it wasn't always that way).

71

For nights at home.

For housing options amid renovation and upheaval.

For architects and contractors who cover for you when your mind   is elsewhere.

For miracle devices and those who implant them.

For 98.6, give or take.

For gains in body weight (J's, at least).

For our church community, our school community, and the countless times you've been there for us.

For today.

For Ode to Joy.

For piano teachers.

For Granny Annie and Nana Mary, may they rest in peace.

For staying in bounds on the Road Hole.

For neighbors who bag your leaves, feed your cat and house your guinea pigs.

For the support of family near and far.

For donors, volunteers, tutors and others who take the time.

For expert care within walking distance.

For doctors who appreciate origami, Ms. Pacman, and pause long enough to show a kid her own neutrophils under the microscope.

For the fact there were neutrophils to be found (490 at last count).

We're thankful today. Hope you are, too. Be well.

I was amazed at J's courage every time she was accessed, though I learned not to show it. *Why are you staring at me?* I was so proud of her, and sometimes I'd tell her. *What's the big deal?* Then, sometimes, *Thanks, Dad,* and she'd grin at me.

She paid close attention, with no interest in easing the reality of what was transpiring, Emla notwithstanding. She participated in whatever ways the nurse found safe and acceptable. If the nurse was new, J's participation would be limited. But CAT/CR nurses developed confidence in J, and though she never was allowed to insert or remove a needle, soon she was sanitizing her skin in preparation and performing her own saline and Heparin flushes. This gave her some control over what was flowing into her veins. Whatever supplies went unused, she'd ask to keep, and if there wasn't a needle or some potential hazard involved, her request would be granted. J began to accumulate quite a collection of hospital supplies.

Many days at CAT/CR were long and tedious. After she was accessed, a small amount of blood drawn, we'd wait to hear her counts. If her counts were high enough, we'd see Dr. Whangbo, Dr. Shimamura or the day's hematology attending, and they'd tell us to come back in another day or two. If the counts were low, they'd order up another bag and we'd settle in.

Children's Hospital regularly broadcasts some troubling event via intercom, color-coded to let those in charge know what the problem is and keep others blissfully ignorant. There was also a regular check of fire security, in which bells and lights went off and doors closed automatically. The emergencies, real and preparatory, served as reminders that all was not well in the building or could be expected to turn at any time. I didn't need the reminder.

As nonchalant as J seemed about all the pokes and transfusions, if I needed to go to the cafeteria, pharmacy or bathroom, she would want to know how long I'd be gone, to let the nurse know and, ideally, to ask the nurse to hang out while I was away. My simple presence was as important as anything I did. Woody Allen: *Ninety percent of life is showing up.*

A truck parked near an intake for the ventilation system and its exhaust was drawn up to the CAT/CR. The smell arrived as a *What's that?* whiff but the fumes grew strong within seconds. J was hooked up to a bag and a pole, making transport difficult, and there seemed to be no clear backup plan to keep her isolated and safe. This played into both of our fears. At which point would the fumes pose risk greater than evacuating into a crowd of people? When does a cocoon become a coffin? But before seeking haven that was less unsafe than where we were, the truck was moved and the fumes abated.

Another day, a breach in the hospital security system caused alarms to sound, and we watched through the window in our door as the immune-robust were evacuated. There was chaos outside our room, serious enough that others were being hurriedly moved, and we were watching from a fishbowl. Should we leave? Into that crowd? Where would we go? The nurse said stay put, and stay tuned. She couldn't tell us what the crisis was, but she was watching out for us. Again, the crisis passed as little more than a test of the staff's emergency readiness. An ominous, anonymous package wasn't ominous or anonymous anymore. From the fishbowl, as the evacuees filed by in return, J asked me to close the curtain.

Neither event prepared us for an otherwise mundane infusion that went terribly wrong minutes before we were to leave for home. J had received platelets, and I had settled into a complacency of assumption that nothing went wrong with an infusion. J had uneventfully received maybe forty bags of red cells or platelets, and this seemed just one more. But as we were thinking about packing up and preparing to leave the CAT/CR, J complained of tightness in her throat, and labored to breathe. Hives emerged. I pushed the emergency button, within seconds a team arrived, and J, petrified, was breathing through an oxygen mask. The problem came and went quickly, because her port had not yet been deaccessed, and intravenous benedryl and Tylenol went right to work. Hives disappeared, steady breathing returned, but we settled back in to make sure that was the end of it, and it was. It also was the last time J would receive blood products without first receiving benedryl and Tylenol preemptively. I watched J's infusions differently from that day forward. *Why are you staring at me?* And I understood on a different level why, should transplant be necessary, minimizing transfusions of the blood of strangers was in her best interest until that day came.

A decision about transplant wasn't imminent, but it was blinking faintly on the radar screen. Though J was maintaining blood for longer stretches, none of her counts were rising in any meaningful way. The neutrophils were teasing us, the hematocrit jerking us around. I hung onto good news with all my might.

Dr. Whangbo stopped to see J on a day when cousin Emily had joined us. Great timing. They got to talking about things like blood counts and neutrophils and how such counts are made, and it was a Friday of a holiday weekend, with fewer people around, and, well, Dr. Whangbo had this idea. She invited J and her cousin up to her lab to take a look into the microscopes used to do all those counts. J had a turn, then Emily had a turn, and Dr. Whangbo explained how to tell one cell from another. Neutrophils are tricky to spot, especially when in such short supply, but eventually, there they were, J's own neutrophils. I got a turn, too, but pretty fast it became hard for me to see. I blinked a few times and restored my composure to its full upright and locked position.

J dictated, I posted: "*Dear friends, Friday is my dad's birthday and we're doing something special but I can't tell you what because my dad's posting this message (I'm telling him what to write) and it's a secret to him. We'll be spending the first part of his birthday at the CAT/CR, but we'll still get to celebrate. I've been reading all of your entries and it really puts a smile on my face. I learned the Nutcracker on the piano (Overture) and it's coming along quite well. My Grandma Joan has a very nice piano, it's from Steinway & Sons, and it sounds terrific. I also get to practice my piano on a keyboard that you can roll up and take with you (to CAT/CR, among other places). I got it for my birthday from my Aunt Mary Jo (also known as Aunt Wrapping Paper because she gives me so many gifts). She's coming from Santa Rosa, California, and she's coming to visit us for a few days before Christmas and for a day or so after. I'm very excited! That's all for now. Bedtime. Goodnight, J.*"

Sometimes the heat in Joan's building would come on with such force that J's room could hit 80 fast. After kissing her forehead, I'd crack the window, and look into the distance at the brightly lit Golden Dome. Under the Dome, politicians were debating who could marry whom in Massachusetts, whether men belonged with men, women with women, and what it all might mean for the institution of marriage. I had one marriage that failed, but my former wife and I crashed and burned on our own, unassisted by same-sex couples. I'm unclear on what our failure meant for the overall institution. I suspect the institution took little notice. Worse would have been the toll on our children, had we had any, but our marriage was blessed in that damage in its failure was limited to ourselves and our beagle.

My marriage to Jody was surviving J's catastrophic illness. Each of us had own own way of maintaining our sanity while remaining attentive and supportive of J and her precarious situation. Over the years of our marriage, Jody and I had learned to communicate well, to listen deeply, and deal with difficult and divisive issues. That wasn't an easy evolution for me, but I got there, learning to hear without taking offense or getting defensive.

J's illness profoundly complicated this communication. As the illness moved from onset to inexplicable fevers to frequent transfusions to surgery to treatment, I needed a way to witness without feeling, to watch as time after time a nurse shoved a needle into her chest and drew out some of her suddenly nonrenewable resource, to learn hard truths and filter them quietly to that place in the mind that holds emotions such as fear with a certain nonchalance. A friend had a name for it: denial. I disagreed. Denial would be somehow finding a way to pretend that it all wasn't happening. I made no pretense that this wasn't happening. I knew what was happening, and there was no comprehending or denying it. I was educating myself daily to understand the illness and treatment without overwhelming my ability to positively impact J's emotional state.

J looked to her parents for a sense of how to react to the chaos that had overtaken her body. I couldn't step outside the room every time something bad happened to her, because something bad happened to her with such regularity, and often I was the only parent there. I needed a means of putting my fears on hold. A way to not scream *Oh, God!* and mirror horror for my child with each new piece of bad news, each new psychic or physical assault. I sought deferral, not denial. I'd take a hard look at it eventually, perhaps with a happy and healthy child to bolster my spirits. I'd get around to it.

This was no way to proceed for Jody, who needed to regularly, if not daily, discuss the emotional roller coaster she was on, to share, to commiserate, to revisit the horrors as a means of making whatever sense could be made of them. An immediate accounting sustains her and helps her to live her life in a difficult time, and such conversation had served our marriage well. But now, it served only one of us well. Jody could only deal with the horrors and be present in a positive way for J if she had a place to go at the end of the day with the heartache and fear. I couldn't be that place. *I can't be there for you in that way and for J in the way she needs me.* This painful truth hurt both of us. Perhaps if Jody did not have a therapist or family or close friends to talk to, I would have found a way to be there for her in that way, but I can't imagine how.

Thank God there were other ears available, other sources of the empathy of which I was depleted.

Jody posted: *"Paul said the best birthday present he received today was news of J's hemoglobin and hematacrit INCREASING. We thought J would need a red blood transfusion today, but the docs said no. This is very good news. It has been 2 weeks and 2 days (and now counting) since she has needed red blood. This is the longest she has gone without RBC since she was diagnosed in mid September! J is happy too. She did get platelets today. It's been a week and 2 days since she has had to have those. And that's the longest period between those transfusions, too."*

I had a growing and ominous sense that the pressure was affecting my judgment. The ordeal of starting the antibiotic dosing pump was one indication. A visiting nurse instructed Jody and I on how to work the pump, and such was the advanced technology behind the instrument that making it work was fairly simple and straightforward. Had it been an MP3 player or a video recorder, we would simply have read over the instructions, plugged in this, pushed that, inserted something else and watched what happened. No big price to pay if it failed. The pump, however, hooked up to our daughter, was meant to push fluid into a manmade reservoir perhaps an inch from her heart, and though the machine was equipped with an idiot chip and therefore smart enough to allow for human error, I was so nervous without the visiting nurse as backup that I couldn't remember the simple steps involved, and Jody wasn't much better. Learning to perform a procedure that, done wrong, had any potential to inflict further harm upon J added a layer of stress I'd never felt before, and strained my capacities and judgment in frightening ways.

The shit hit the fan, almost literally, at the end of an outpatient day at the CAT/CR. If this wasn't the day of J's allergic reaction to blood products, it was near that time. Joan was out. I spent time after returning with J from the hospital pouring a mix of hot water and Arm & Hammer Super Washing Soda into drains that had been backing up, including J's toilet. The problem had come and gone for days, been attended to but not resolved by the super and plumbers, and was freaking me out. A unit on a lower floor in Joan's building had sewage from who knows whose apartment spill out into their living space. They were livid, and they weren't even immune suppressed. So far, the fifth floor had avoided that extreme, a perk of elevation, but we were living in a building where the toilets were backing up and spilling their contents onto the floor. I didn't have to check with the doctors to know the risk inherent in this. I yearned to be back on Seven West, and felt an urgency to fix the problem or consider telling another of Jody's parents their home was somehow not clean enough and moving yet again. But where?

Dad had taught me the hot water and washing soda solution, and it had been my one fool-proof act of plumbing for many years in many homes. You pour the liquid into the toilet or basin and use a plunger to work it into the clog. Often the problem clears quickly and the drain empties following a few burps of relief. Turning on the hot water and letting it run a few minutes completes the process. Sometimes the clog needs two or three treatments to clear, and sometimes the clog stubbornly demands a professional. But never had it reversed flow.

I brought this limited and risk-free plumbing skill of mine to bear on Joan's apartment, and after a few treatments of soda and hot water and extensive plunging, there was burping and bubbles from within, and then there was movement. Another bucket of soda and hot water, a bit more plunging, and the water flowed freely. With a great sense of relief and accomplishment, I turned on the hot water to complete the process, watched it flow down the drain, and I ran down the hall to check on dinner.

Indeed, while tending to the plumbing, I was cooking dinner. I don't recall just what I had in the oven, probably J's favorite garlic roast chicken, but within minutes I was in Joan's bathroom calling to Jody to bring towels and come help, and for J to stay far away. The water was surging back through the drain in Joan's shower, filling the low basin, spilling out onto the tile floor and into her bedroom.

The super, a tolerant and understanding man with a short history of dealing with the building's toxic personalities, patiently explained that the problem was much bigger than a clog and that when the water got flowing from one apartment in the century-old building, then was met with a surge from a lower apartment, the effect could be to change direction. *Oh*, I said, wringing out a towel. I apologized. I felt like a fool, and the feeling wasn't fleeting. I can still summon it up, no problem. J, Jody, and Joan were more forgiving of me than I was. All I knew was, I needed to get myself together, and defer multitasking to more a settled time. Which, I told myself, would surely come.

Professional plumbers arrived and did what they could to address a major systemic problem. They didn't ask for my help, and I didn't offer. Soon, water and waste consistently flowed in the direction intended, and without stopping to visit the neighbors. I focused on appointments, meds and meals, one at a time.

Jody posted: *"I'm a bit discouraged. Two reasons: 1) J's blood counts inch up ever-so-slowly. Even though this is normal and she is doing quite well (according to the doctors), I was hoping she'd go back to school in early January. She is still immuno-suppressed. She still gets blood transfusions. They are fewer and far between, now, but she has also been having mild allergic reactions to the platelets. That is frustrating. And sort of scary for her. But the doctors and nurses are really on top of all this, so I know it will sort itself out. 2) I was looking forward to celebrating Christmas in our newly renovated house. This is no one's fault but my own, getting my hopes up. My aunt and uncle have been working their butts off to push the project through. It is just bigger than we thought, at first. We haven't slept in our own beds, in our own house since the first week in June."*

I investigated paints. In the new normal, with environmental toxins among possible culprits, I couldn't take chances with the renovation. I discovered the acronym VOC, for volatile organic compounds. I'd never heard of them before, but in addition to greatly improving paint quality, VOC give off fumes hazardous to a fragile body. I discussed them with my house painter, encouraged the use of low-VOC paints, but we discovered low-VOC paints aren't great when exposed to moisture, like, say, in a bathroom. They don't hold up as well to weather and sun. And they weren't available in colors darker than pastel. So I did more research, and determined that most standard paints, exterior and interior, are thought to lose toxicity pretty fast. We chose paints that would last where needed, with low-VOC where possible, and figured the fumes would delay our return home another week or two. I found a good low-VOC alternative to coat the new cork floor in the kitchen and sunroom, one of the few renovation-related jobs I did myself. *On your knees, boy.*

Uncle Dave learned of a company specializing in cleaning air ducts. We signed them up. The counter installer handed me a can of some nasty thing he said I should apply to the granite. I read the contents, did a little research, and stuck the unopened can on the shelf till the next time Brookline had a day for dumping toxic substances. When that day came, I was out of town, and I've probably still got the can squirreled away somewhere. But it's not on the granite. Nobody's inhaling it.

The super in Joan's building got serious about renovating his basement apartment. The fumes and dust wafted up to the fifth floor. We opened windows, turned on fans and put on sweaters. I checked the humidifiers again. It's amazing how fast mold grows in those things.

At least we could count on yoga to be safe. Lucy had arranged for a yoga instructor to come and work with J once a week. Yoga Peggy knew the rules about symptoms, was conscientious, and her sessions offered an important break from the sedentary life we were living. A bit after the fact, I told Dr. Whangbo about it. She decided yoga was fine, except if J's platelets were low, when extreme positions might cause problems. Yoga became more meditational on low-platelet days.

J posted: *"Let's talk about Christmas. I had a great one. My aunt Mary Jo came to visit and we got her a bagpipe for Christmas. We bought it while we were in Scotland last summer. She loves it. It has a green covering with gold tassels. We also gave her a McLean crest to be stitched onto the cloth. She already plays the piano and other instruments and works with a children's chorus. Today we went to CAT/CR at Children's Hospital and I didn't need a transfusion. That's a very good thing. Today I went to my grandparents' house in Brookline and made a movie with my grandma's video camera. The movie involved a disco lamp. It also has advertising for Purell and Trader Joe's. It's very funny. I had a very good time making it. That's all for now, J."*

Though we never determined the cause of J's illness, genetics were ruled out, which led us to pursue the immunosuppressant treatment. The goal was not cure, but transfusion independence; that she could make enough blood to get by, though her counts might never approach normal. In about 70 percent of aplastic anemia patients, there is enough positive change in the immune system to consider the response to this treatment sufficient. J responded initially, but her counts plateaued well short of safety.

Early on, my brother-in-law Nicola, a scientist, found a German study that showed when response to initial treatment fails, a second go-round of immunosuppressants often achieves a satisfactory response. We expected this, but J's doctors instead said we should proceed to transplant. This development was head-spinning. Transplant was last-ditch. We weren't last ditch yet, were we? And yet, the numbers teased, but they didn't lie. The counts were so clearly insufficient.

Statistics meant little to me – what good is a 70 percent success rate when you've already landed in the bottom 30 with a disease that affects two in a million? I also was becoming aware that most studies involving significant numbers of patients reflected findings that were years old. The studies were the most recent vetted and published information, the best *proven* science, and yet given the pace of contemporary science in the study of stem cells, a few years old seemed grossly out of date. Understanding in this area, though slowed by political and moral opposition to the particular form of stem cells known as embryonic, was progressing at such a rate that we needed to look, not backward, but forward. Mortality rates that went back 10 or 20 years reflected understanding of transplant that was archaic. Given the condition of the blood supply, a child with aplastic anemia receiving 80 transfusions in the late 1980s essentially traded one disease for another – hepatitis, AIDS, maybe both. The numbers that came to really mean something related to transplant timing: that engraftment is more achievable and complications more manageable when the transplant is done within a year of initial diagnosis, the sooner the better, and when transfusions number fewer than 100.

From the moment J was first diagnosed, her grandma Lucy worked the phones, beginning to connect and differentiate how aplastic anemia was understood and treated in Boston and elsewhere. Europe had vastly different approaches to transplant. So did major pediatric centers in the U.S. But there was some consensus. All of them would want to give ATG and cyclosporine at least one chance before moving to transplant. And all agreed: *Time is of the essence.* I heard that phrase many times, but I recall the first. It was Lucy. Then she had to get off the phone, because, well, her mom was dying.

Jody posted: *"Paul and I both felt so restored, attending church today. Not only is it the church that we have been attending since before J was born (and where she had her naming ceremony), it is truly a second home for all three of us (third home? fourth home?). Needless to say, we are not back at 50 Oakland Road yet. People always ask us for an estimated move-back-in date. Paul came up with a good response: "2006!" Susan and Kate Culman came over and J and Katie threw dried soup beans at each other. I love it when this apartment is full of the sound of giggling girls."*

I loved that sound, too—J giggling with another child, a cousin, an aunt, a grandparent, or more often by herself as she listened to Eric Idle as the army general recommending strategy to the president in *Charlie and the Great Glass Elevator: Let's blow them up first, crash bang whallop bang bang bang bang bang. Come on Mr. P, let's have some really super duper explosions.* And then as the president's nanny and vice president: *Silence you silly boy.* There are other sounds I associate with Joan's apartment: the whistle and clang from the radiator as the heat came on; the neurotically clicking electric pilot on the stovetop; the alarm as I fumbled with J's antibiotic doser; Joan's voice on the message each time we waited to pick up for fear of telemarketers; the siren call of the burbling plumbing; the exasperated neighbor asking me, *What are you doing up there?* Other, more pleasing sounds emanated from the living room: Mary Jo and Julie double-teaming J on a piano lesson; another pianist friend bringing some joy and accompanying caroling; Mary Jo, no longer with a parent to care for, playing like I hadn't heard her in years, and storytelling in her trademark multidirectional stream of consciousness; Joan practicing her own licks on the piano and picking up her fiddle to duet with J; and J practicing. J's playing was beginning to take my breath away. I'd never heard Ode to Joy so full of meaning. For all isolation excluded, it didn't lack a soundtrack.

We prepared for the news. In this transitional juncture, we were blessed to have Akiko Shimamura to explain, to hold our hands, to assess the gravity of the situation and give us reason to hope. And so we listened closely as Akiko explained why she was unconvinced by research indicating a second round of ATG and cyclosporine held significant promise. The marginal movement in J's blood counts, which we clung to as a sign of something positive, provided no real reason to hope. Transplant, Akiko said, provided that hope.

Jennifer Whangbo was with us that day, as well, and she brought a stack of printouts chronicling the course of J's treatment—counts and transfusions, in particular. Nothing in the numbers was positive, not the ANC that approached 500 before falling back, nor the decreasing but ongoing necessity for platelet and RBC transfusions. We were far from transfusion independence. The social worker Christine, of Make-a-Wish fame, was there to provide support at the revelation of difficult news. Jody took the news hard. There was so much risk involved in transplant. As Akiko described the conclusion she had come to, and Jennifer cited confirmation in her printouts, Jody's hope absorbed a potent blow. I was too oblivious or deadened to react that way. *Just the facts, ma'am.*

J was already at about 60 transfusions as we met, and even if we put the transplant process in motion immediately, she would have 80 when she received the new stem cells. Better, Akiko advised, that we proceed to transplant, especially in light of the many good donor matches available to us. We were lucky, she said. There were donors for us. That is not always the case. These strangers possessed the potential for cure.

Akiko said the Children's/Dana-Farber approach to transplant was conservative and that we needed to be aware of work going on elsewhere. She didn't recommend the alternatives, but she wanted us aware of them. In a position such as we were in, regrets are inevitable. We needed to know what others were doing.

The Reindeer Collision

By J

One Christmas Eve when all the people of Boston were asleep Santa came with his reindeer to town. But by accident he let go of the reins! Oh no! All the reindeer fell because without the sleigh they could not stay floating. So they fell and they landed in San Francisco! Plus they landed on a very pointy building and got pricked on their butts! Then they slid down the top of the point of the building and landed on the Golden Gate Bridge. But they were very confused because they thought the Golden Gate Bridge was gold, and it was red! So they dove into the water and got eaten by sharks. When Santa heard of all this, he was very angry! He called the cops to get the reindeer but then the cops got eaten by sharks too! By now Santa was furious! He himself went to find his reindeer, but he was eaten by Jaws! But Jaws found Santa so chubby that Santa made a clog in his throat and Jaws died and that is why Jaws has never been seen anymore. By now you may be wondering did Santa live? Well. Santa managed to squirm out of Jaws' mouth but still he has a lot of scrapes from Jaws' teeth. That is why nobody sees Santa. He doesn't want you to see all of his scrapes. The end.

CHAPTER FIVE

Know Where to Go

Hematopoeitic stem cells are extraordinary things, they're virtually life itself, and make it seem that bone marrow transplant ought to go by another name. With transplant, I think of a surgeon cutting open one body, removing a malfunctioning organ and replacing it with one from another person for whom, whatever the reason, it was expendable. The attention to detail that goes into this type of transplant is so vital, and must be meticulous if there is any chance for it to work. The new organ must be placed precisely and stitched securely into its new home. The organ can do none of this itself. Without human hands to guide it, the organ will just sit there until it expires.

With a stem cell transplant, the meticulous work is in the divination of a donor, preparation of the recipient, then in the delivery of the marrow and subsequent aggressive marshaling of a sort of detente between the cells and their new host. But the actual transplant is a mere infusion, much like any other bag of platelets or red cells hanging from the IV poll. The stem cells arrive in a beer cooler. They drip from a bag through a catheter line and into the body through the preferred man-made access point, and once inside, they know where to go. They do not need a surgeon's guidance, or some cellular GPS for negotiating their strange new home. The doctor isn't even in the room the whole time, leaving most of the transplant work to the nurses. The stem cells go straight to where they're needed, begin anew their duplicative process and get to work delivering, nurturing and healing. They won't know whether they'll be welcome. They may in fact be ornery on arrival in their new environs and need doctors to help negotiate that. But they simply know where to go.

We, too, as a family, would know where to go when the time came. Striving to be meticulous, our work was in comprehending the stakes and possibilities, preparing J and choosing where and in whom to place our faith.

When we thanked Joan, packed up and moved back into our own home in late January 2006, we knew we wouldn't be there long.

Jody posted: *"Grandma Lucy and I are just back from a whirlwind, two-day, fact-finding mission to Seattle where they know a lot about treatment of aplastic anemia. Paul stayed in Brookline with J. We are still in the process of deciding what the next step will be. We'll let you know as soon as we can. Meanwhile, J continues to look decidedly NOT sick, bouncing around our "new" house and playing with all the toys and crafts that have been packed away since last June when we moved out. Today, Paul caught two salamanders in our yard for J to look at (she can't touch or keep them). She was EXTREMELY excited. We are so happy in our home."*

When the veneer of security fails and the chaos begins to swirl about you, it's good to be near experts in the field of assessing chaos and illuminating the path forward. When the chaos is the sudden onset of a child's life-threatening illness, there is perhaps no better place to be than Boston, where so many great hands, hearts and minds of pediatric medicine practice. So I considered it a blessing, and always will, that when J's body began its inexplicable revolt, we lived within walking distance of Boston Children's Hospital. The early days and weeks of her hospitalization are a montage of vivid and searing moments, none more deeply carved into my psyche than the night, in the Emergency Department, when a doctor probed into J's nostril with what appeared to be a long wooden matchstick, seeking to stop the flow of blood by cauterizing what her own body hadn't the platelets to stop itself. It worked. The bleeding stopped. It was the first of many times when J saw her parents turning to the doctors of Children's Hospital to do what we could not. We relied on those doctors and nurses for so many things, not the least of which was keeping J alive. J developed a profound trust in them.

I was largely ignorant of blood's components and what they do, and yet I found myself in conversation with men and women of staggering intellects and passions and strategies for healing, and I was desperate to understand what they were saying and why they believed what they believed. The doctors expected this of Jody and I, and soon. Decisions needed to be made. Some doctors were quite good at explaining things at my comprehension level, but others were not, and faced with the responsibility of decision-making and my daughter's life at stake, I couldn't afford not to elevate my understanding. I needed to comprehend what was being pumped into her and why. To see why it was a good thing for a child who couldn't stop bleeding on her own to have her chest intentionally cut open for installation of an artificial reservoir of blood. If I couldn't see it, how could J?

Jody, with her Ph.D. in clinical psychology, had less catching up than I did, at least with regard to her ability to comprehend a scientific paper, but both of us educated ourselves in a hurry, pestered our doctors and nurses for more information, and then explained to J as best we could the need for the surgeries, the meds, the pokes, and the incessant invasions of her privacy. I remember stressing to J how smart and talented these doctors were, how we needed to place our faith in them. And yet she ultimately didn't have a say into whether she underwent surgery or what went into her body orally or through an IV line. She would somehow need to accept such unfair and powerless realities, and all the ambiguous facts, as there were many more to come. But I believe she achieved a remarkable understanding, or at least acceptance, of the chaos that had erupted in her body, and though she is unlikely to ever comprehend the unfairness, she came to place her faith in and deeply trust the doctors and nurses at Children's Hospital. She knew they were keeping her alive, that with time we might put this struggle behind her, and she was grateful.

And so it was not easy to explain to her why we were leaving home and the doctors and nurses she trusted so, and moving cross-country to Seattle.

More than once, Akiko described the Boston approach to transplant as conservative, the doctors proponents of the tried and true. Also, more than once, Akiko said we would need to educate ourselves about different and experimental approaches elsewhere. Transplant for aplastic anemia was evolving, amid varied research, much of it promising but unproven, much of it contradictory. She wanted us to know about all of it so we could make an informed decision.

Months earlier, Lucy began researching different approaches to transplant and assessing what would be best for J. She had become, in essence, an advocate for J, a role that grew in importance to me the further into the journey we went. No patient should be without an advocate. There is much at stake, and the fog is dense. Lucy was uniquely qualified for this role, not merely because of the intensity of her feelings for J but because of her resourceful nature, intellect and her access to leading minds of medical science. Early on, Lucy planted the seed in both Jody and I that if transplant became necessary, we might need to consider leaving Boston. Though there was uniformity in initial treatment of aplastic anemia, that was not the case with transplant, where the differences were significant. There might even be cause to leave the country.

The pediatric doctors of the Dana-Farber Cancer Institute form the oncology/hematology team at Children's. In winter 2006, when transplant had become our only option, their approach was to treat aplastic anemia much like certain cancers, with a reliance on high dosage irradiation in combination with chemo drugs to set the stage for the transplant. The process is called conditioning, and the purpose is essentially to wipe out the immune system and prepare it to start from scratch. Sometimes the transplant is done using the child's own stem cells, but that isn't possible with severe aplastic anemia. There simply are no cells to start over with. A matched sibling can simplify the process, and allow for conditioning of lesser toxity, but we would require an anonymous and unrelated donor.

In this case, the conditioning process additionally prepares the body to accept the foreign cells. The more smoothly this goes, the better. Perhaps the greatest risk during transplant is from infection, because if the patient's immune system wasn't suppressed by the illness itself, then the conditioning process knocks it down, and prepares it to receive the new marrow. To have a second chance, the immune system must start with no fighting chance of its own.

To the degree that it is understood, and treatable, aplastic anemia has cancer research to thank. The disease is rare and remains more mysterious in origin than known, with research funding that is comparatively paltry, and yet treatment is effective largely because the immune deficiency that defines it is so similar to the immune suppression demanded in treating leukemia and lymphoma. And though there are differing styles and approaches to treatment, there is no great difference from one major treatment center to another in terms of the ultimate bottom line: mortality rates. From City of Hope to Sloan-Kettering, the efficacy in treatment of aplastic anemia is quite similar.

Transplant success requires that the donor and recipient are compatible, *histocompatible*, which is determined by microscopic examination of shared genetic qualities. Along with their understanding of histocompatability, transplant doctors have greatly improved the chances that the donor stem cells will begin to grow and make new blood cells. The donor cells are the graft, the recipient the host, and the two don't get along naturally. So while waiting for engraftment, controlling infection and managing graft vs. host disease (GVDH) become crucial to success of the transplant. Much of this is addressed in transplant preparation known as conditioning, and the Boston approach was to rely heavily on radiation. In this, they were not alone. The approach at Sloan-Kettering was essentially the same. It is known as myeloablative transplant, in which doctors count on days of intense total body irradiation to wipe out the recipient's immune system so it won't reject the new cells. This remains a vital therapy in transplants for leukemia, and no doubt will for years to come. Its proponents referred to conditioning with less radiation as a mini-transplant, which made it sound to me like a cute idea but not a serious option.

But J didn't have cancer, and in the course of better understanding our options and what was best for her, we became aware of a trend: research institutions increasingly were moving away from the reliance on irradiation to prepare an aplastic anemia patient for transplant. One doctor said, *Why ablate what's already dead?* In essence, the disease itself has wiped out the immune system, and so taken care of one aspect of the transplant conditioning. Some research institutes had cut way back on use of irradiation in transplant conditioning, others had abandoned it altogether. Lacking a consensus, it was clear to us that heavy reliance on radiation had in many places become counter-prescribed for severe aplastic anemia.

Boston didn't buy this approach and considered it experimental and unproven as with Campath, I'd let go. They saw the radiation as a major contributor to their success in achieving engraftment and controlling GVHD. Some patients transplanted for aplastic anemia later develop leukemia or another blood cancer known as myelodysplastic syndrome, and Boston believed those possibilities were better dealt with at the time of transplant, even for those with no evident cellular disposition toward the cancers. While aware of the ongoing research into low-dose irradiation elsewhere, Boston said there had not been a study of sufficient size and scope making a strong and sufficiently vetted case on the pages of the journal of the American Society of Hematology. Boston wanted to see proof written, quite literally, in Blood.

That would have comforted us, as well. But the more Lucy and Jody uncovered in interviews, and the more I read, the more I came to believe there was no such published study as yet partly because aplastic anemia was such a rare disease, a hematology orphan lucky to find a foster home among the oncologists, and partly because the various hospitals performing transplants for aplastic anemia did so largely independent of one another, even those using the same conditioning regimen. As a result, there was no big picture of what was working. The independents touted their own successes, and left it at that.

But this was changing rapidly, and we were in the midst of the change. The various and growing practitioners of the Seattle protocol were coming together in a collaborative sharing of numbers, and soon would be producing results of research studies with a significantly greater and more compelling number of participant patients.   I had no interest in taking chances with our daughter's treatment, but first Jody, then I came to feel that the Boston approach was frustratingly reluctant to give credibility to the advances we were hearing and reading about elsewhere. We seemed to be seeking cure amid profound change that was lapping the tried and true. But what if we were wrong?

As I gather my thoughts to write about this, it seems clear-cut and obvious, a revisionist byproduct of retrospect, but it was mind-boggling at the time, and I was slow and even reluctant to get it. We lived in an unbelievably supportive community of family and friends, within walking distance of some of the great scientists and medical practitioners and one of the preeminent cancer and hematology institutes in the world. The

Jimmy Fund, the pediatric wing of Dana-Farber, is well-funded, widely known and respected for its work and cutting-edge research. J still had a fighting chance because of this good fortune.

I was counting my blessings, and so many of them wore M.D., Ph.D. and Harvard Medical School on the nametag. They'd become my safety net, and I was reluctant to leave and take my chances—J's chances—elsewhere. Vetted science was with us. Geography was with us. We had the best doctors anywhere taking care of J. The conservative approach was attractive to me. *First do no harm.* And yet.

Was it in J's best interest to wait for the vetted and published research to catch up? Might it be better to take a chance on that progressive research at transplant's pioneering home? This wasn't desperation and laetrile in Tijuana. And the hope versus risk equation seemed increasingly weighted in favor of hope.

I had been slow to join Jody and Lucy in the research. Blunt conversation about mortality and toxicity and strongly made but conflicting arguments threatened to destroy my shield and set my Jesus eyes to blinking. So Jody and Lucy began the difficult work without me. This soon felt cowardly, though, and I joined in.

My sense that the transplant paradigm was shifting went on like a light bulb in a cave. We were riding a wave in the midst of a sea change, and had to choose. They all wanted to save J's life—the doctors in Boston, the doctors in Seattle, and the doctors around the country and beyond who got on the phone or exchanged emails with Lucy, Jody and I. I was coming to believe that a decision to have the transplant in Boston would be based on our fear of something bad that might happen later. Leaving for Seattle filled me with hope for all the good that might happen later. It was a hope based as much on faith as vetted science, but I was blessed with a belief that, either way, I would have my daughter with me for some time to come. J would have a future. How much of a future, how full a life, could we give her? That's what the choice came down to.

Had I been a single parent, without all the resources, human and otherwise, available to me—especially without Jody and Lucy's tireless research—I would have simply trusted the system I was in, been grateful for the help and perhaps learned after the fact what might have been possible elsewhere. I wasn't a single parent, though, and I had unbelievable support in coming to the right decision. For all our differences in coping style, Jody and I were a team, and our purpose was clear. Lucy shared that sense of purpose, and it carried she and Jody through extensive, excruciating interviews and research into toxicity and mortality. It carried the two of them to Seattle, where fact-finding and site visits essentially sealed the deal, producing a clarity I'd never have found on my own. Lucy did much of the research, and so much to make sense of it. She revealed her findings in our living room in an afternoon of raw honesty and awe and draining emotion, exhilaration and hope. She brought a Buddhist singing bowl. The resonant hum of the gong gifted the three of us with a mutual place to gather our spiritual senses and settle the manic whir in our heads.

I was astounded by the willingness of experts in transplant not directly involved in J's care to take my calls or respond in detail to my emails. My experience at Boston Children's told me just how busy with matters of life and death these people were. And yet, with so much at stake, complete strangers willingly helped us. The Aplastic Anemia & MDS International Foundation connected us to sources and resources. The Be the Match national marrow donor program put me in touch with the Center for International Blood and Marrow Transplant Research in Wisconsin, which put me in touch with directors of transplant at hospitals in Northern California and England. The British doctor exchanged emails with me, addressing several questions. The Californian got on the phone with me and, though pressed for time, was eager to help. It's an unusual position to put doctors in, asking for advice on a patient they'd neither seen nor familiarized themselves with, but provided the basic information of J's case—diagnosis of severe aplastic anemia, failure of initial treatment, transplant called for—the recommendation to avoid high dosage radiation was clear.

Jody and Lucy met and spoke with many others. We gathered the information and shared it. The head of transplant at a Midwestern hospital told Jody from his cellphone driving home late one night that his facility recently had switched from high-dosage radiation, the same protocol as Boston, to no radiation at all. He'd leap-frogged Seattle. J didn't need *any* radiation, he insisted. This was the direction European transplant was headed.

What was enough and what was too much? This was at the heart of our quandary, and the contradictions were many. We would never resolve them all, and I struggled to determine which questions mattered and which I could let go of. I called the office of the head of pediatric transplant at a major university hospital in the South. The doctor's secretary took my information, and soon the doctor called me back.

In a frantic and confused state that was no doubt familiar to her, I explained our situation. First she defused my obsession with the drug Campath, which had been stressed by the British doctor as an alternative to ATG. *It wouldn't be harmful,* the Southern doctor said, *but it's not necessary.* But then she replaced it with a question I'd not had. She said a key question in choosing a treatment center would be whether it readily had access to defibrotide. *Not all have access to it.* It was the first and only time I had heard of defibrotide, a recently developed anticoagulant used in the event of occlusive disease of the liver, a life-threatening concern in transplant. Boston had led the research into it, but as with Campath, I let go of defibrotide as crucial to our decision.

The Southern doctor further recommended that we choose a facility with a strong pediatric focus, with nurses dedicated to transplant and able to deal immediately with issues unique to pediatric transplant as they come up. She said in that respect Boston had everything going for it—and here she was preaching to the choir. And though she never quite said this, I heard: *There is no reason to look elsewhere, aside from the TBI.* In this, she was in agreement with the London doctor: *We feel it is important to avoid irradiation, especially in young aplastic anemia patients.*

A trusted doctor, speaking out of his area of expertise, had told me the toxicities of irradiation and chemo drugs were so similar that I shouldn't get too caught up in assessing which was the lesser of two evils for J. I decided he was wrong. In fact, much scientific effort was going into minimizing the use of both. There was no consensus to be found, but the clearest trend for aplastic anemia was away from irradiation. The Northern California doctor said his facility was in the process of adopting the Seattle regimen, and that this was the trend in transplant for aplastic anemia. He wished us good luck.

Even Dana-Farber/Boston Children's was listed as a test site for the Seattle regimen, though it was not clear when they might begin participation. It wouldn't be with us.

Each conversation I participated in produced a bit more clarity as well as information I hadn't expected. But we would never reach a point of perfect clarity, devoid of ambiguity. The fog would never lift, not completely. Still, the fingers pointed away from high dosage radiation. Outside the circle of our immediate care, that's all we heard. After fact-gathering from major transplant centers around the country, Lucy created a spreadsheet comparison—with numbers of pediatric transplants performed, amount of TBI used in conditioning, other aspects of conditioning, mortality rates, etc. Most had adopted, or were in the process of adopting, the regimen developed and being advanced in Seattle.

Research papers on transplant and severe aplastic anemia all seemed to emanate or cite studies from Seattle, and one name in particular stood out: Joachim Deeg, a German doctor attracted to Seattle for its work in transplant. Rare was the study of transplant and aplastic anemia that didn't at least cite the work of Deeg and colleagues. There was a history of bone marrow transplant in Seattle dating to the 1950s, a history of Nobel laureates, and a current generation of doctors who continued to advance expertise in the area we so desperately needed it.

They were testing the chemo fludarabine as a means of lowering reliance on the higher-toxicity cyclophosphamide, the predominant chemo drug in use. They weren't using Campath, and hadn't jumped on the no-TBI bandwagon. Seattle's research on lowering reliance on TBI went back more than a decade, and the amount settled on was a single dose of 200 sonogray. Enough, they determined, but not too much.

For pediatric care, Boston is as good as it gets. We knew that. We'd benefitted from it. But we had become convinced the high-dosage radiation was unnecessary, and Boston offered no alternative. *Why ablate what doesn't exist?* There was no indication of cancer in J, and doctors in Seattle saw no reason to expect there would be. Although J's T cells might have been up to no good, there seemed no need for a scorched-earth approach to getting her body ready for its foreign invasion. *Why ablate what doesn't exist?*

I hung up the phone, and shook. We had to move again.

Jody posted: *"We have decided that we want J to have her transplant in Seattle at their Children's Hospital/Seattle Cancer Care Alliance. We carefully compared the treatment protocols used in Boston and Seattle, consulted with many aplastic anemia experts all over the country, and came to this decision. We feel really good about it. We wish we didn't have to leave Boston Children's Hospital—she has received and continues to receive excellent care there. The decision was very specifically about comparing the medicines each hospital uses in unrelated donor bone marrow transplants for kids with aplastic anemia. We will miss J's doctors here very much and look forward to returning to Boston Children's for her ongoing care. As you can imagine, these last few weeks have been emotionally exhausting. It is a relief to know, now, where we are headed."*

My change of heart was gradual, but it felt jarringly sudden to Jody. One day I told her, *We're going to Seattle.* I didn't mean it as the final word, or as an edict, but merely as a clear statement of where I stood. This was always going to be a consensus decision. It had to be. Regrets were certain no matter what decision we made. We had to be on the same page. But I caught Jody by surprise. She was distrustful that I could shift so suddenly in a matter of such gravity. Jody had made the fact-finding visit to Seattle with Lucy. They conducted exhaustive and excruciating research before I jumped in. And yet Jody wasn't ready for the way I ended my personal struggle with such clarity. In truth, I felt at least as much ambiguity as clarity, but such was the position I found myself in.

Lower-radiation transplant was available at hospitals closer to us than Seattle, and we considered some, notably the University of Minnesota, where a family friend had taken a child to successfully treat a nasty cancer. The strong pediatric focus made Minnesota worth considering and interviewing, but not enough for us to visit. Fairly early, our choice became between Boston and Seattle. Once convinced of the merits of lower radiation, we chose Seattle because it was the transplant pioneer, performed more transplants and had more experience with transplant for aplastic anemia. We knew that Seattle's focus was all ages, not specifically pediatrics, but that the transplant itself would be performed at Children's Hospital Seattle, a modern and vibrant facility that impressed Lucy and Jody. Jody, especially, had been spoiled by the nurses in Boston. Perhaps it was Seattle's nurses who sealed the deal.

The decision made perfect sense, and there was no looking back. But we needed to tell J.

Although I felt more strongly than ever that J should have a say in as many decisions about her care as was reasonable, Jody and I didn't involve her in where the transplant should take place. That was way too much for a child, even one who'd already proven she could handle a lot of pain, uncertainty and changes of address. To the best of our ability, we didn't conduct our research or have related conversations in her presence. She was just settling and finding some peace and security in her newly renovated home, and sheltering her from the stressful decision seemed the best way to go. But once we had decided, we would tell her immediately, explaining why we were moving, that we would all be together the entire time, what she would be undergoing and that we strongly believed this was best for her.

Bone marrow transplantation was pioneered in the 1950s and '60s by E. Donnell Thomas, who would earn a Nobel Prize for his work. To read about those early transplants is to be reminded how fortunate we were to live in a time when there was more than a long-shot treatment. Early transplants were frighteningly experimental, and the question of what made a donor compatible was barely understood.

The very idea to employ irradiation for pre-transplant conditioning was frightful in origin—coming when scientists such as Thomas and Rainer Storb learned of human immune systems shutting down in the weeks following the dropping of the atomic bomb on Hiroshima. Somehow an intellectual link was made between the atom bomb's ablation of human immune systems and paving the way to a new system and a second chance for leukemia patients.

I latched onto the names in Seattle—Storb, Deeg, Woolfrey, Sanders—well before I actually met them. I talked by phone with one pediatric transplant specialist there, Dr. Paul Carpenter. He'd been helpful with Lucy's fact-finding mission. Generous with his time, he put my mind at ease on a number of topics. Still, we hadn't left Boston yet, and already I missed Drs. Shimamura and Whangbo and Shannon. I didn't know a single Seattle nurse yet.

But it was time to tell J. We sat down in our sunroom, in the shade of a towering oak, next to the vacant space where her beloved guinea pigs had once resided and by the TV we'd recently spent hours watching Olympians Irina Slutskaya and Johnny Weir perform their dervish spins.

J knew something was up. Jody did most of the talking. She's reassuring, clear, and chooses her words with great care. We explained that to cure her disease, J would need a bone marrow transplant; that the best place in the world to have a transplant was in Seattle, so we were going there; that the Boston doctors were telling the Seattle doctors all about her, and that the Seattle doctors were probably going to use the donor that Boston had found.

J wanted a better explanation of why we had to leave, and we offered one as best we could. Then she asked if she'd have to have chemo, and we said yes. The news hit her hard. *No! No! No!* She asked why several times, but she never asked about radiation. Images of her own baldness at once shoved her violently into a future soon to come and transported her back to Seven West, with its bleeding lips and gums and yellow bags on IV poles and nurses in splatter-proof garb and collapsed veins and clumps in the tub and nothing-tastes-good meals.

J was inconsolable. But Jody and I sat with her and told her we'd be with her the whole time, and the upset passed in time, and as she gathered herself she made Jody promise to get her lots of wigs. Soon she was on the phone with her Aunt Kristin, matter-of-factly saying we were moving to Seattle, that she was going to have a transplant and would lose her hair.

Maybe that night, maybe a day or two later, Jody and I sat at the dining room table with J and Emily, playing a game spontaneously invented for the occasion. Moving clockwise round the table, we made up sentences that began with whichever letter of the alphabet arrived when it was your turn. The game was a hoot, and the sentences became goofier the further into the alphabet we went. We got to Y. It was J's turn. She thought for a moment, and let the sentence come to her: *Yeah, I'm going to be cured!*

My brother Steve came to visit from Michigan. He is a chiropractor known for his healing work. J was excited, and flattered, that he came especially to work with her, and I was moved that he would make the trip. She basked in the adjustments and energy work. Steve adjusted Jody and I as well. After two quick days, he was packing again and J and I were loading into the car to take him to Logan. After putting his bag into the trunk, he didn't notice my hand as I bent to assist J with her seatbelt. The hatch slammed down on my finger, and I howled in pain. Steve quickly opened the hatch again, releasing me, and as I hopped around holding my right angle of a finger and muttering *Ow Ow Ow,* though J remembers me yelling *Fuck Fuck Fuck,* I tried to reassure J that it was nothing serious. My Jesus face was failing me. J looked terrified. Steve apologized, came back inside with us and got me some ice to apply to my throbbing digit. We called Steve a cab. Jody came home and insisted I go to the emergency room for an X-ray. The ER, complete with loud and belligerent drunk, was worse than the injury. After several hours, the X-ray showed nothing broken, so there was nothing to be done but wait for the healing, and hope I'd brought nothing infectious home from the emergency room.

Daily during our abbreviated return to our renovated home, J spent hours in the new window seat, listening to stories on CD: various tales by Roald Dahl and E.B. White, which could not have been more different; the adventures of Harry Potter and Geronimo Stilton, a mouse whose incessant cheese jokes were working some dark curse worthy of Hogwarts and turning my head to gouda. While she listened, J created. She'd draw, sew, make crafts, create worlds with her Legos.

Before the renovation, there'd been a solid wall where she sat, but Aunt Linda's redesign pushed that wall out nearly five feet, installed seven windows, and created a southeast-facing space naturally lit for much of the day. The transformation was extraordinary, and J was drawn to it immediately. It wasn't designed specially for a kid in isolation, it just worked out that way.

There were many people we wanted to see before leaving for Seattle, but I was getting particularly paranoid about contacts. I got sick of hearing myself say no, but I wanted clear sailing to Seattle. An infection could screw up everything, and so I became adamant about limiting visitors. But whenever I'd get adamant, Jody and J would start working me.

I had to admit, J got so much from seeing her cousins, and her Aunt Kristin had a rare gift for brightening J up just by walking through the front door. The Moscufos were all healthy. So I said OK, they can come over for dinner, and it was one of the more wonderful evenings I've ever spent. Nicola, Kristin, Michela and Emily brought so much joy into our home, and the evening ended way past the kids' bedtime with a goofy coronation ceremony. Loud squeals and shrieks and laughter transported J miles from the shadow that hung over us. Such a gift, such a blessed evening, for her to experience such joy with people she loves so completely.

The next day, it was just J and me again. J was enjoying the sunlight in the window seat, playing Legos, and I was in the kitchen, washing dishes or maybe fixing her a meal or preparing another pile of skunky pills to smack down T cells. There was no longer a wall separating the kitchen from the dining room, but she was in her own world, and began to sing: *Can I do anything heroic?* I don't know where the words came from. I'd not heard the words or the tune previously, and haven't since. *Can I do anything heroic?* They were original, I supposed. She repeated them over and over, chantlike. *Can I do anything heroic?*

Then she glanced up, stopped her chant and caught me looking. *Why are you staring at me?*

Jody posted: "*Spoke to the bone marrow donor search coordinator in Seattle on Friday and they said they will probably use the donor that Dana Farber found. He is a 28-year-old man in the USA. I keep trying to imagine him. Surely he has a halo. Or at least wings. Anyway, this means that they will likely schedule the transplant very soon. It will probably be a date in late March and we will need to be in Seattle within three weeks from now. That is great news because it is hard to wait. Now, if I could just get all the boxes unpacked before then. Paul and I and J had our first weekly (we hope) Family Writing Hour this morning. J is such a good writer and we want to encourage it more. So we all sat around the breakfast table in our pajamas and we each wrote a scene for our new play, "Fish to Minnows and the Great White Shark." It's hilarious. A triggerfish (Jody) won't let the a fisherman (Paul)*

catch her until he learns her real name (a multi-syllabic Hawaiian name).
The Great White Shark (J) saves the day. Twice. (Note to my colleagues: no
fair psychoanalyzing.) One of the co-ministers of our church visited Friday
and helped us brainstorm ideas for a healing circle/service being planned for
J. "But how am I going to get the healing?" J asked me. "I can't be there. Oh,
I know, you could put the prayers in water and then I can drink the water!"

I had mixed feelings about the healing service. I liked that it provided a time and a place for the extended support community following our journey on the Carepage to come together spiritually if not all geographically. Even for our many friends not inclined toward prayer, this was a good thing, as it provided somewhere to go and something to do with their concern for our daughter. So many were following our ordeal through the Carepage.

What made me wary was my own faith, an odd hybrid of cynicism and wonder. And what would it mean to J? We had friends and family who sought God's intervention on J's behalf. But if God was going to get involved in solving the problem, what role did he have in its cause? And while intervening for J, what about those other kids on Seven West for whom the prayer was no less fervent? They weren't all going to make it.

Mom infused water with such power—Lourdes and Fatima water, especially, helping the cripple to rise right up out of that chair. That was her top-shelf holy water, hidden away for occasions. The everyday holy water came from our neighborhood church, where even our simple parish priest could with a simple blessing turn the water holy and somehow transformative, though its powers were diluted in Mom's mind because the Virgin had never appeared at its source. Sometimes Mom would enlist Dad's help and they'd drive the narrow and serpentine Pasadena Freeway to the little church next door to Dodger Stadium to fill up a jug. Mom was sure the water that flowed from Father Thomas's tap was full of mystical potential. Something of a Lourdes Lite. I knew it had fluoride in it, coming as it did from an L.A. tap, but wasn't sure of the rest.

Mom always kept holy water on a table by the front door. Two ceramic Siamese twins held poles with small bowls at their tips, suspended by string. Inside the bowls were moistened squares of sponge. Whenever I'd leave home, Mom tried to make sure some got on my forehead, a blessing made by her index finger in the shape of a cross. I don't know what it accomplished; she did. To keep a child safe and protected, to ward off evil, a parent does what a parent can. To avoid this soggy ritual commemorating Jesus' crucifixion, I learned not to call out that I was leaving until the oak door was closing behind me.

Years later, whenever J or I would be leaving the house, especially in the summer, Jody would come running with the SPF-30 or above. It had to be strong to keep us safe from the sun's rays. SPF-15 was like the water from the local church—limited power, better than nothing. Jody'd get mad when I'd start laughing, but I couldn't help it. It was just too ironic not to laugh. Jody understood the irony, but didn't laugh. Melanoma killed her stepdad. The house where she religiously applied the SPF had been purchased with inheritance from him. We wouldn't have afforded it otherwise. A parent does what a parent can.

I never figured myself for performing ritual and dispensing liquid protection by the front door, but here I was, back in the foyer of the renovated version of the home made possible by Jody's late stepfather, turning away most who came knocking but allowing some in. The ones granted admission were asked to take off their shoes, and then I'd ask them to hold out their hands, and I'd squirt Purell.

I posted: *"There are a number of friends we've made at Children's Hospital/Seven West with whom I keep up-to-date via their Carepages. Their ups and downs help me keep our own journey in perspective. And while the successful donor search has filled us with hope for J, there's a young woman currently at Children's who is not so fortunate. Amelia Quinn is in great need of a transplant, but has no match in the national pool. For a month or two her family and friends have organized events to seek a match, without success. They're trying again this week. There is a bone marrow drive in the Moot Court Room of Northeastern Law School this Thursday and Friday from 10 to 5. From Amelia's mom: "I would like everyone you know to know about this. And everyone in your company, and everyone in your church, and everyone at your school. I want EVERYONE to know about this drive. We still don't have a match, which is okay, but I'd like to take advantage of the opportunity given us by NU to register as many new donors as possible."*

Due in part to my doubts about the efficacy of prayer, I intended to let Jody attend the healing service while I stayed with J. Jody wanted both of us at the service, but I worried J would feel left out. She couldn't be in that crowd, and I wanted to be both places. Lacking bilocation, I opted for being with J, even after a number of people volunteered to stay with her. But then the yoga instructor, Peggy, someone with a recent history of doing healing work with J, volunteered to be with her. They'd do yoga and meditate, or maybe just hang out and play a game. So I went.

We gathered in Lyon Chapel, a century-old space at its best early in the day, when sunlight illuminates the woods outside and streams though tall, clear windows, creating a place of peace, beauty and wonder. But the day had gone dark as friends and family, adults and children, filed inside. Cousin Myles, whom J had met hours into his first day on the planet, took it all in from his mother Rachel's arms. There were perhaps a hundred people there. In a dark space lit by candles, I sat with Jody and tried to keep it together. For the most part, I succeeded, though I was moved by the concern and support. My friends were cutting through my defenses. I saw a minister from another church who'd opened my eyes to the benefits of Revs. Martha and Jim's co-ministry; hobbled by a recent fall, the minister would be diagnosed with Lou Gehrig's Disease while we were in Seattle.

One member of our congregation played piano, another performed a modern dance. Lucy made a video of J explaining yoga poses, and Kristin projected this onto the wall, which brought a vital and robust-looking J to the service in a powerful way. Rev. Martha asked me to choose readings, and I suggested options from the Gospel of Thomas, taken from the Elaine Pagels book. There's something about an apostle remembered for his doubt that resonates strongly in me, though the words of Thomas that I chose were about faith and human connection to divinity.

On CD, John Hiatt sang "Have a Little Faith in Me," which Jody and I had danced to at our wedding reception. Springsteen sang: *I've got a date, I can't be late, with all that heaven will allow.* We listened to Bach's 2-Part Inventions #4 in D-minor, a piece J was learning. If healing is getting to a place of gratitude and possibility, then healing took place that night. A calling out of names brought ancestors to the ceremony. Rev. Jim led a processional in which, one by one, all in attendance poured water into a communal bowl. Afterward, Rev. Martha poured the water into a star-shaped bottle, and packaged it to go, which J had requested as a means of delivering *healing energy* to her.

Jody left for home immediately to get J ready for bed. I stayed at the church and heard thanks for allowing the service. I muttered something incomprehensible in reply. When I returned home, J splashed a few drops of the communal water on an itchy arm, and soon said the arm wasn't itchy anymore.

Jody read to J and put her to bed, but I stopped in to say goodnight. J and I had an evolving ritual for saying good night that involved competition for which of us loved the other more. *I love you SO much.* We borrowed from "Toy Story." *I love you to infinity, and beyond!* Sometimes we'd retrace where we'd been. *I love you all the way to San Francisco, then on a bus across the Golden Gate through Marin County to Santa Rosa, and back.* Back and forth we'd volley in our testimonial tennis match. *I love you across the Bourne Bridge, around the Cape Cod Rotary, to the Woods Hole Ferry, across the Sound to Vineyard Haven, over to West Tisbury and down the dirt road to Grandma's.* It became hand-over-hand up the baseball bat, and J thought she had me defeated with *I love you googleplex.* Sometimes she would go for the quick win: *I love you more LA LA LA LA I CAN'T HEAR YOU!*

I wouldn't be defeated, and found my googleplex trump on the eastern coast of Scotland. *All the way to Fife.*

Fife is a mystical place, for no better reason than the existence of a golf course. Duart Castle isn't in Fife, but Saint Andrews is. It is where Old Tom and Young Tom posed for their Southern California early bird special coffee shop portrait. Dad and I were intent on playing the Old Course before life and the end of it wrecked that plan. But he was so present that morning with the Germans.

All the way to Fife, I told J, and bent to kiss her forehead.

And beyond! J replied, smiled and closed her eyes to seal the victory.

Akiko wrote: "*To Whom It May Concern: I am the hematologist caring for J McLean, an eight year old girl with idiopathic aplastic anemia. She had no hematologic response to ATG (anti-thymocyte globulin) and cyclosporin.*

Since she has no siblings, the only curative therapy for her aplastic anemia is a hematopoietic stem cell transplant from an unrelated donor. Unrelated donor transplants carry higher transplant-related toxicities than matched sibling donor transplants. Her family would like to pursue a reduced-intensity conditioning regimen that has been recently described to minimize potential toxicities. Although long-term data are still limited, it is also possible that long-term problems, such as solid tumors, might also be lower with this regimen since it uses reduced doses of radiation. This regimen is not currently offered at Children's Hospital/Dana Farber Cancer Institute. The Fred Hutchinson Cancer Research Center has experience with this treatment and is a leading center for this regimen."

The letter was written and sent, with another from David Scheff, J's pediatrician back in the old normal, to Tufts Health Plan in hopes they'd cover the transplant if we went out of state. I feared they'd deny it, but the insurer took little time to respond that it would cover the transplant in Seattle. With clear and to the point letters, Drs. Shimamura and Scheff came through for us again.

Health insurance never added to the chaos of J's illness. This is high among our blessings. A few years earlier, after I'd left my job and its health insurance, Jody spent a year post-grad at MIT, and we were covered while she was there. Then that position ended, we were left to our own devices, and our own devices weren't up to the challenge. We decided to save money on insurance and went with the only catastrophic coverage we could find. We had the policy for a year. Filing a claim was complicated and bureaucratic, the company didn't seem to be doing anything other than accept our payment, and soon we started to hear and read bad things. We'd made a bad decision, and we felt vulnerable. So we decided to bite the bullet and buy first-rate health insurance.

We decided on Tufts. It was expensive, but we breathed easier. Then J became ill, and the last thing we needed was to deal with heartless bureaucracy. We didn't have to. The coverage was good and the company so efficient that we felt no burden from matters related to insurance. We didn't need insurance headaches, and we didn't have them. Were we unable to afford such a policy, ours might be a very different story. We counted our blessings. There were more than we could count, and more by the day.

We had to figure out how to get to Seattle. The last place a kid with no immune system should be is on a crowded commercial airplane. We'd kept J without a fever or a sniffle since November, we'd entered transplant mode, and we couldn't risk exposing her to that sweating, shivering presence in 27B. We'd heard about corporate alliances with jets that get sick kids where they need to go, and we contacted them. We were eligible, but there were limits to how far they'd fly us, and we'd need a backup plan—and possibly have to board a commercial flight after all. We looked into a private charter—about $40,000 to Seattle. I told Jody we should find a commercial red-eye flight midweek and enlist the flight attendants' help to keep ourselves as separate as possible. But that still left too much to chance.

Unbeknownst to us, a family at our church had some history and experience with medical complications and travel. Commercial flights had long ceased to be an option for them, so they'd joined what amounts to a private jet time-share. They'd followed our story on the Carepage, and one of their children suggested that they donate the flight to us. The parents liked the idea. I was humbled by the generosity, but nothing surprised me by now. Somewhere there was a twenty-something human being a few weeks away from undergoing a procedure to extract—to harvest, though bone—a significant amount of marrow to give another chance at life to someone he or she did not know.

J posted: "*I'm excited about Seattle because on the plane it's really comfortable it seems like and they have lots of food that you can order. And my grandma's coming on the plane with us and my aunt Mary Jo's going to visit twice. I don't care very much that my hair is going to fall out, as long as I get to see my guinea pig afterwards and my cat and go back to school and see all my friends. That's all for now. Bye from J.*"

Jody found a house sitter. We said goodbyes and accepted good wishes. We booked rooms for ourselves and Joan at the Residence Inn on South Lake Union, just down the hill from the Seattle Cancer Care Alliance. We didn't expect to be at the Residence Inn for long. We were third on the waiting list for a two-bedroom apartment at the Pete Gross House, a residential building devoted to SCCA patients and families, with a school on its first floor.

J and I made one last trip to CAT/CR for a transfusion; one for the road. The nurses threw J a surprise party. Dr. Whangbo prescribed an antibiotic to take with us, just in case J spiked a fever in transit. She wished us well and said she looked forward to our return. It was comforting to think we'd return to her care in a few months. Her role in getting us to this point was immeasurable.

After the appointment, J talked me into taking her to Seven West to say some goodbyes. This would entail a long walk through the corridors of Children's, but we'd been there long enough to know the back way, apart from the crowds, and to take the more lightly travelled elevators devoted to patients. It was strange walking back through the doors, after applying Purell, of a place that had been so attentive to our every need but now had other individuals and more urgent matters to concern themselves with. The nurses were busy, and getting their attention wasn't easy. Mostly drive-by smiles and *I can't talk now*'s and *I'll try to find her*'s.

Nurse Jenn was on duty, but we couldn't find her right away. At Seven West, you don't go knocking on doors. We poked around. I checked to see if I still knew the code to the kitchen; I did. Most of the patients and parents were strangers to us. We hadn't been in-patient for about four months, and there'd been lots of turnover, good news and bad. We went to the activity room to check on Ms. Pac-Man and saw the familiar faces of Linda Ireland and her son Roy. Linda was talking with Wallace Quinn, and she introduced me. I told them we were off the next day for Seattle. *Did we have a donor?* Wallace wanted to know. I told him we did. I knew from their Carepage that his daughter Amelia had relapsed, needed a transplant and was without a match. J tugged on my arm, we wished them well, and continued our search for Nurse Jenn. We found her, and J got the hug and photograph she wished for. Then we said goodbye, Jenn responded to a ringing bell, and we headed toward the door. Passing the resource room, we spotted Jacob Noddy and his dad playing cribbage. We waved, and left.

The next morning, we loaded up the Quest, a hand-me-down from Gerry and Lucy with a dashboard ganesh, and left for Hanscom Air Force Base and our ride to Seattle. Gerry went with us, to see us off and drive the van home. There wasn't room for Lucy, but she sent us off with freshly made turkey clubs from Sealey's, J's favorite neighborhood diner. At Hanscom, I spoke our identifying info into a box, the gate opened and we drove in. Another gate opened and we drove right onto the tarmac. The pilots greeted us. They would be the only other people on board. We jammed bags into every available space, and climbed aboard. We were airborne in minutes.

We stopped to refuel in St. Paul, Minnesota. Had we placed greater value on pediatric focus than on transplant experience, we might have unloaded our bags there. Instead, we stepped out onto the frigid tarmac to stretch our legs, and in minutes were back on board and headed west.

The views were spectacular, increasingly so the further west we flew. Then there was Rainier dominating the horizon in the distance. We cleared the Cascades and approached Seattle from the north, taking in Puget Sound and the city on descent. Jody pointed out the Space Needle to J. Joan pointed out the Olympic Peninsula. I looked for the Kingdome, where as a sports writer I'd watched the Lakers and Sonics meet in the playoffs before about 40,000 people a quarter-century earlier. The Kingdome was nowhere to be seen. It had been razed. Two new stadiums stood side by side, one for the Mariners, the other for the Seahawks, who'd just lost the Super Bowl. Things had changed. I wasn't looking for a crowd of 40,000 to spend time with.

I posted: *"J and I, the early risers, viewed the new dawn over Lake Union from the sofa of our suite at the Residence Inn. The transformation from darkness to light and anticipation of a new day reminded J of standing in Aunt Wrapping Paper's kitchen in Santa Rosa, California, in the early morning hours and peering through the window of her room to see if the light was on yet. Sometimes we'd wait for the light to come on, sometimes we'd just barge right in. Aunt Wrapping Paper always said that was OK. She lets J get away with anything. She'll join us in Seattle in a week or so."*

CHAPTER SIX

Living in a Post-9/11 Flight Pattern

W e had a room with a view of Hooters. Among a restaurant row, multimillion-dollar yachts docked and awaiting an offer, and a massive parking lot, Hooters was the most neon distraction from our Residence Inn suite. Beyond was an expansive northwesterly view of Lake Union, Queen Anne Hill, the distant Aurora Bridge and Gasworks Park.

It takes but one flight into Seattle to know this to be a city set amid stunning natural beauty, of which the bright and colorful sign for Hooters would not be one. Jody, Joan and I shared a laugh, J wanted an explanation of what was so funny, and I said it seemed funny that a restaurant would have such a name. She wondered what the name meant, and I said it was a reference to the prominent breasts of staff, that this was a restaurant that had adopted those breasts as its very reason for being, that it was like calling a restaurant Boobs, and she agreed that this was an odd thing to name a restaurant. She still didn't get what was so funny, but we moved on.

Our latest home was new to J and I, but Jody had visited with Lucy weeks earlier on their whirlwind tour of housing, transplant facilities and mortality rates, and so had a sense of things. She directed our attention to the view from J's room, which faced east, up Aloha Street two blocks to the SCCA, rising like a crystal cathedral. This was where we would go for appointments. This was where our hope was now kept.

Jody's previous visit didn't prepare her for the plane. She was startled right along with J and I, first at the mysterious sound of the engine on approach, growing steadily louder, then the sudden and jarring emergence into view, coming within inches of the Residence Inn rooftop, or so it seemed, as it swooped down like an osprey fixed on its catch, leveling like a pelican at the last minute and touching down with a soft splash amid the kayaks, water taxis and sailboats on Lake Union. We'd somehow dropped into a freakish post-9/11 dream, with planes strafing our home but never quite colliding.

Seaplanes carried tourists to views of Rainier and the Cascades. They took traffic reporters to survey rush hour. They flew commuters to or from the islands of Puget Sound. They took off and landed multiple times daily and reminded me of trips with my parents to watch the mail arrive by helicopter next to the par-3 golf course where I'd learn the game. Mom would sing her helicopter song, rhyming land with band to the tune of a Souza march or reasonable facsimile. I didn't sing along.

The sound recalled helicopters flying in formation in the middle of the night, dropping malathion to confront fruit fly infestations in my early 1980s leafy LA suburb. We were told to stay indoors during the spraying, to keep windows closed, and trust that the government knew what it was doing. I'd lie awake and the sound of the choppers would transport me to Hollywood, to *Apocalypse Now* at the Cinerama Dome and napalm's smell of victory in the morning. Vietnam films were as close as I got to that war. I was in the last draft lottery, and was never called.

After the malathion spraying, my Datsun 210 would be spotted with a yellow goo, like New England pine pollen, only stickier. My throat would be tight, and I'd invariably awaken with a headache.

After awhile, the seaplanes of Lake Union ceased to startle. I learned to recognize the low muffled sound of the approach, growing steadily louder, and I'd go to the window in the kitchenette or living room to watch the plane burst into view. Later, after we'd left the Residence Inn, I'd take in the landings from the living room or roof deck of our apartment. The planes appeared to land so near the kayakers and other boaters, amid such nonchalance. J and Jody bored of the landings. I never did.

We'd been met at Seattle's Boeing Field by two new friends, Barbara and Ann, who didn't know us but learned of us through a mutual friend, followed our Carepage story, and adopted us. They brought one car for the luggage and another for the people. They chauffeured us to the hotel, then to the market and helped us track down misplaced luggage, requiring a return trip to the airport. They brought J a bagful of goodies and Seattle adventure coupons to be redeemed by Barb and Ann at times of J's choosing. J was touched. Barb was a veteran of transplant and the healing process at the SCCA, and a volunteer at Seattle Children's Hospital; she and Ann quickly established themselves as people who couldn't do enough for us. Our Seattle community was fast forming. With our anonymous donor, friends arranging flights, and now Barb and Ann, our list of angels grew daily.

On our first full day in Seattle, we had no medical appointments. This would not soon be repeated. I rented a car, and we saw some sights.

The Residence Inn was popular with SCCA patients for its proximity to the sprawling campus of the SCCA/Fred Hutchinson Cancer Research Center. Guests were invited to a buffet each morning, and J was eager to check it out, but she was banned from the fingered foods of any buffet. The place had an indoor pool and spa, but they also were off limits to J. Just before her diagnosis, she'd taken to swimming in a big way. Now she hadn't swam since that steamy solarium pool in the North Sea town of Nairn. She couldn't wait to dive back in, and she was jealous if Jody or I went for a swim or a soak. She was jealous, too, if one of us went to the buffet. She pleaded, and Jody thought maybe it was OK, but I went straight for the veto. J was not wading into that crowd or eating food with mystery fingerprints. I accepted her dirty look as well deserved.

At the breakfast buffet, minus my family, a bald woman in a head scarf gave me a knowing smile. I don't know if she knew what she thought she knew. My shaved head was filling in, and I assumed she took this to mean we were kindred chemo spirits. Maybe she was right. My spirit, at least, was kindred. I smiled back and then sat down with my bagel and complimentary Starbucks and read a *New York Times* review of James Reston Jr.'s memoir of his daughter's illness. That got me to wondering how and when I would lift my blinders on J's illness. It also made me not want to read anything like that for a while. Joan Didion's "The Year of Magical Thinking," about losing her husband and daughter in close succession, was on the best seller list. Such a gifted writer, but I didn't dare read it.

I missed Drs. Whangbo and Shimamura and our Boston nurses. I didn't know the SCCA people yet. I had no doubt about the care offered at the SCCA, about the expertise in transplant, but they weren't our doctors yet. Our doctors were across the continent. Seattle wasn't even my time zone yet. J complained about the low back seat of the rental car.

Our second morning, J greeted us with the suggestion: *Let's watch the sunrise,* and we saw the blue waters of Lake Union come to life. The day was busy with tests and appointments at the SCCA. I began to meet the doctors and nurses I'd entrusted with J's care and would rely on into the summer. Trusting without knowing requires a leap of faith, but what I did know was these were the people other transplant facilities looked to for support and direction. If I had to leap, this was the place to land.

I wrote down names, not counting on an already bad memory maxed out trying to tell fludarabine from fluconazole. I wasn't alone in struggling to keep track of drugs. Even the SCCA computer network at some point confused ambizome for ampicillin on the list of what J had an allergic reaction to; we corrected the record on a recurring basis. I jotted down Debbie the transplant receptionist, Dow the physician's assistant, nurses Melissa and Monica. I didn't need to jot down the larger-than-life Jean Sanders, a name I already knew as a pioneer who had seen pediatric transplant through the bleak and into the promise. She still heard from a forty-something transplanted as a teen.

In our get-acquainted, get-started session, Dr. Sanders had a stubborn cough, apologized for it, assured us she was past contagious, and got to business. She went over the Boston chronology we knew well—date of diagnosis, initial treatment delayed by fevers, failure to respond, number of transfusions, allergic reactions—and told us about the science behind histocompatibility and our donor match.

While we reviewed the records, J grew wary of the persistent bark, and gave me *that look* several times. I enlisted my eyebrows into a don't-worry face. If anyone knew not to come to work sick, it was Jean Sanders in Transplant. I trusted that. J didn't. New place, new face, new rules. Her own faith was still in transit from the Northeast to the Northwest, and the new doctor had a cough. In Boston, she'd have been wearing a mask or not been there at all. *Why is this OK?*

J was in transition. We all were. All three of us attended appointments. That hadn't been the case in Boston, not for months. We also were hearing a different kind of advice from what we were used to. We had lunch in the SCCA cafeteria, within the safe confines of our care and with our doctor's OK. This would not have happened in Boston, where J's regular pediatrician came to visit one day, apologized for his sniffles, wore a mask and never actually stepped into our room, only cracked the door enough to say what he needed to say and find out what he needed to find out. Now J, in a strange city, sat across a table from a new doctor who coughed and said not to worry. In the back of her mind, chemo loomed. *What are we doing here?*

The day's appointments went so efficiently, and I wondered if Radiology would again play spoiler. That answer would have to wait till another day, but we didn't wait 15 minutes for an appointment all day. When we did wait, it was in the Transplant Clinic lobby, where J spotted a table with built-in chessboard. She'd been teaching me how to play. The set was missing a piece, so a pocket Purell became a pawn. After a few moves, our name was called, I pocketed the pawn, and we finished up in Transplant with Monica and Dow, went over the next day's schedule, and went on our way.

J and I raced to the elevator button. She won. We waited for the elevator, and I checked out the portrait looming over the hallway: E. Donnall Thomas. I vaguely recognized the name. He was why we were in Seattle, but I didn't know that yet.

The routine of reviewing J's daily meds schedule with nurses continued in Seattle. Prescriptions and doses were adjusted with such regularity, it was important to check in multiple times weekly on whether our lists matched and she was on the right stuff. They usually did.

The best news for J was that she could stop taking cyclosporine. And she could resume brushing and flossing her teeth. For months she'd relied on soft sponges and rinses to clean her teeth, as aggressive brushing and flossing were thought to put her at risk of infection. The SCCA reversed that. Infection risk, the SCCA dentist said, was greatest when the teeth and gums were neglected. Hearing this, J shot me a quizzical look. After one visit with the SCCA pediatric dentist, J was brushing and flossing gently once again. *I've a feeling we're not in Kansas anymore.*

Jody posted: "*We are impressed by the efficiency of the Seattle Cancer Care Alliance clinic and the Children's Hospital Seattle. All the facilities seem brand-new and uncrowded and streamlined. The medical team here does not require J to wear a mask when she's out and about. They emphasize the hand-washing instead. That's taken some getting used to because J feels more comfortable with a mask on. Here, when you wear a mask, it means you have a cold or something and are trying to prevent YOUR germs from spreading, instead of vice versa. I feel like we're getting all our R&R in, gearing up for transplant. J will have day surgery on March 31 to take out her port-a-cath and to install a different catheter. On April 1st, she will be admitted to the hospital to start her chemotherapy. Her transplant is now scheduled for April 6th. This is her namesake Grandpa Gerry's birthday!"*

April 6 was also the day my dad died. An eventful date.

Before we left for Seattle, J had been aching to play in the snow, and it was a lousy year for it. Winter 2005-06 was frigid but the snow didn't amount to much. J had an unusual amount of time and freedom for snow play, but mostly we had ice and bitter cold. When it finally snowed, enough to create a sled run on our lawn, she and I bundled up and got right to it. J had so much fun. The old wooden sled I'd rescued from a church rummage sale didn't build up all that much speed sliding down the mild slope of our lawn, but it was enough to make stopping short of the rock wall at lawn's edge difficult. So we built up a mound of snow at the edge of the lawn, and I shoveled until I'd created a reasonably soft landing on the sidewalk should the mound not do the trick. Now she could go right down the hill and smack into the bank to stop.

I helped drag the sled to the beginning of the run, and she waited for me to get back to the bottom, so I could play backup to the mound and catch her as needed. I think she liked me in a role of making things OK. I know I did. Down she came, howling with delight, time after time, especially this one time as the sled got a little out of control and tipped over and she rolled into the snow. She wasn't wearing a helmet. She was relatively low in platelets. And right as the sled was tipping and J tumbling off, along came Gerry and Lucy for a surprise visit.

Both appeared shocked, and gave me a disbelieving, *What the hell are you doing?* look, and I knew why. Had the roles been reversed, I would have been frightened and angry. This was not smart. It was fun, but it was not smart. But when it was just the two of us, left to my judgment, the risk of injury felt limited and acceptable, and J was all for it. No doubt my decision was fueled by my hunger for feeling I could make her safe, and I was sick of telling her no. It felt good to step out of my conservative, voice-of-caution role. When I stepped back in, it became that much harder to draw me out.

Across Fairview Avenue from the Residence Inn, on the south shore of Lake Union, a small park with a play structure beckoned to us. J and Jody wanted to check it out. *There are no kids around,* Jody said in an attempt to reassure me and cut through my reluctance. *No kids NOW,* I clarified with a bark. What about ten minutes ago? What prolific booger picker three potty visits removed from his last brush with soap was swinging from the monkey bars ten minutes ago? We were so close to transplant, we'd not had a fever in months, and I was paranoid or obsessed or some hideous hybrid. Still, I caved. Two to one. This could be made safe. We brought along Purell and went in search of some fun. Saying no all the time can feel like bad medicine.

I posted: "*We're in high spirits today. J got two infusions (which is what these wacky Left Coasters call transfusions), so you know J's bouncing off the walls. Jody and me, too, because we met today with a woman named Christy Satterlee, whose job it was to do the science and find our best match. And so we heard our best description to date of the anonymous person stepping forward to change our lives. We had thought a 28-year-old man had been chosen, but since J has the unbelievable blessing of many potential matches, Christy was able to look a bit further and has found this 25-year-old woman from somewhere in the US who is not only turning her own world upside-down to make her schedule work for us, but is said to be excited to be a donor and is truly as "perfect" a match as an unrelated donor can get. There are no guarantees in this journey, but today's news has filled us even more with hope. We will be able to communicate anonymously with our donor at first. Then, after a year, unless the donor wishes to remain anonymous, we can communicate directly with her, perhaps even meet her. I do hope that will happen. We also learned more today about the conditioning research protocol J will be participating in, and it only made us more hopeful.*"

Seattle, with its extended periods of gloom and drizzle, has a reputation for sending vulnerable psyches into deep funks. One in three Seattle residents, I read, has at least a mild case of seasonal affective disorder, or SAD, and that matched the ratio in my household. But as we settled in, spring was near. Seattle recently had experienced 27 consecutive days of measurable rain, just short of a record, and there'd been another wave of gloom in the days before our arrival. But the sun came out when we arrived. When the sun comes out in Seattle, no pale face wastes the opportunity. Melanoma rates are said to be higher than anywhere.

If I'm depressed, Jody's not. If Jody's depressed, I'm not. I don't know why this is, but it's always been the way with us. We can be contented and happy at the same time; it's been known to happen. But aside from the early days of J's illness, I can't think of a time when we've both been depressed, and there are few things in this life the two of us are more aware of than tendencies toward depression, our own or others we love. I winter in a cave with my light box and one eye on the forsythia buds. Jody tends more toward the talking cure. But when the gloom descends, it's one or the other, never both. There have been times where the rotation has been virtually tidal in its consistency, and reminded to me of California's calendar-based gasoline rationing in the 1970s—her tank hitting empty on the even days and mine the odd. So predictable were we that we'd joke about it.

Doing better, honey?
Yeah, thanks. Your turn.

Words are not always necessary for one to acknowledge the other's emotional state. Simple eye contact is sometimes enough to know. You see it in an expression, sense it in a sigh, hear it in the crinkly opening of another dark chocolate wrapper or the muffled pop of a California Shiraz.

This pattern never made any sense to me; it's simply a fact of our relationship, and one we've been well served to be cognizant of.

Nothing altered this pattern until J became ill. If ever there was a time for both of us to be depressed, that was it. Those early days, it didn't take much to send either of us over the edge. And yet, after the initial time of shock and darkness, I couldn't take my turn. I couldn't afford to be depressed, not unless I wanted to risk dragging my daughter down with me. Depression never felt like a choice before that, and doesn't now, but at the time I banished it. No doubt Jody and J would beg to differ, but I forced consistency upon my emotional state. Hell, if J could accept the severe terms of her indefinite isolation, I could park my darkness for a while—become the boy in the emotional bubble. My blinders effectively negated the pattern of emotional role-switching with Jody; the jetty I erected altered the normal arrival of low tide.

Not that we were altogether without a pattern of role switching. It merely lessened in frequency, changed from depression to influence of fear, and played out most clearly in the decisions regarding where and with whom J could be.

Jody was most concerned with J's emotional state. I focused obsessively on her physical health—symptoms, appointments, meds. When Jody and I did switch roles for reasons of convenience or availability or fatigue, vigilance was compromised and a price was paid, almost always by J. So I focused mostly on those directives that could be traced back to the doctors and their helpers, and found that following them to the letter was the way to go. But out of this role grew the horns of devil's advocacy. I became the family scaredy cat, as J pointed out with some frequency.

In my lifetime, western medicine's understanding of and approach to how the severely immune suppressed should go about their lives have changed drastically. I shudder to think of J in a plastic bubble for months, cut off from all non-medical human contact, all risk, while doctors crossed fingers for a safe re-entry. A parent had little or no access to the child during treatment. That was a millennium ago, and more or less yesterday.

There is no aplastic anemia pandemic on the horizon. This is a wonderful thing. As a result of its rarity, aplastic anemia is in many respects an orphan, a disease that does not command the resources devoted to understanding and treating it of, say, cancer and AIDS. This can be terribly isolating for the "lucky" ones, those for whom ATG/cyclosporine "solves" the problem. Hospitals with doctors who understand the disease well are relatively few, assumptions that it's cancer are common, and the "relief" that it isn't cancer can feel insensitive. And yet this orphan disease shares such infection risk and symptomatic aspects with both cancer and AIDS that advances in research for the latter two have enormously affected the life expectancy of a child or adult with aplastic anemia.

In my lifetime, severe aplastic anemia has been transformed from quite likely fatal to merely life-threatening. With antibiotics, antivirals and other manmade defenses, there are ways to manage symptoms. The Seattle doctors were eager to get J on Bactrim, to guard against a form of stomach pneumonia common to AIDS and transplant, but J had a reaction to it. They thought so highly of the drug that, had there been time, they would have weaned her onto it. But there wasn't time, so another drug developed by AIDS researchers was prescribed. So was Ursodiol. Its inspiration: bear bile. Scientists got wondering why bears don't experience organ failure during hybernation; it's the bile. The orphan benefits from rich cousins and victims of earlier wars.

All of this new hope and better treatment didn't invite disregard for risk but left room for consideration of the bounds of J's isolation. She didn't have to live in a bubble, and yet she couldn't be in any crowded or enclosed space with sick or symptomatic people. But what was acceptable risk? Where did regard for J's emotional state cross over into enemy territory? Where was the line?

A generation of science and medicine tested desperate victims of cancers and AIDS and considered strategies and failed and succeeded and so developed drugs and other means of treating symptoms and side effects and the infections and blood disorders that threaten a life. All of this had created new hope for cures or control of illnesses, and lifted the bubble. What was left outside this reliably safe but drastic measure, this literal protective shield, was trust and interpretation and judgment, and collaboration among doctor, nurse, parent and patient.

In the bubble, there was no balancing physical and emotional well being. Solve the physical problem and, if you're lucky, worry about emotional repercussions later. Outside the bubble, and in a time when even a neutropenic child is more rapidly returned to the parent's care, emotional and social needs are allowed into the healing, which brings the parent's judgment into play along with the doctors' confidence in that judgment.

In this, I never achieved a competency or a consistency, and never fully trusted my own judgment, and so tended to cling to the umbrella of conservatism. I felt safer there, and it came to be expected of me. When I stepped out, it was warily welcome to J—*Are you sure?*—but unnerving to others. Indeed, when I loosened up a little, Jody was likely to jump into the void and becoming the devil's advocate herself.

In Boston and in Seattle, though, there was this consensus: The greatest infection risk was from J herself. And since you can't very well isolate yourself from yourself, you do what you can to stay clean. As this reality set in over time, we evolved toward an awareness that there was no possible way to avoid risk—each dash through the Children's lobby to the CAT/CR served as a reminder—and that we must do what we could to ensure a safe environment. The longer J's immune system was compromised, the more normal this became, and the more matter-of-fact became the daily decisions over what was acceptable and what was not.

When J would have a playdate, it was easier to see the joy than the risk, and heartening for us to see her have fun. She also gained our confidence with her attention to clean practices and avoidance of risky behaviors, in or outside the home. She grew weary of my daily monitoring of her temperature, and other violations of privacy, but she also accepted, and on some level appreciated, that this was my role in the process of her healing. She was as likely to ask, *Aren't you going to check my temperature?*, as scold, *I TOLD you I didn't have a fever!* The line between necessary and neurotic isn't always clear.

Through the six months of J's treatment in Boston, we lived as a role-swapping traditional family, with me having primary responsibility for the home and childcare and Jody maintaining her professional life to some degree, though the demands of J's illness forced her to postpone psychoanalytic training. In these roles, we found a routine and relied on it as we constructed something resembling normalcy. In anticipation of moving to Seattle, Jody created a network of colleagues to work with her patients, and closed her practice.

Moving to Seattle threw us into a new chaos. Together much of the time, both parents available 24/7, the definition of our roles lost its clarity. We could afford to let our guard down more, and that took practice. We had no real priorities other than getting to the transplant in the best health possible. That focus helped transcend the chaos, and it became an extraordinary and unique time for the three of us, bringing us together in all manner of ways.

But the transition was challenging and awkward. I was used to being the primary caregiving parent, but now we could share and I had to figure out how to. This was a great thing for Jody, ending an insane time when she'd somehow have to put concern for her daughter aside to focus on her patients, then switch roles again when the work day was done. But in some ways it was easier for me to take it all on; delegation and sharing of responsibilities leave room for error. Assumptions are dangerous. In the transition, things slipped through the cracks, and failure to pay meticulous attention to detail could and did leave J vulnerable. Jody and I needed to communicate better and somehow get on the same page with regard to the details of J's care. We began to hold daily "rounds."

The Left Coast doctors and nurses turned the Boston approach to keeping J infection-free on its head. A prominent sign in the SCCA lobby instructed people with symptoms to wear masks and directed them to an isolation area. Most days at the clinic began with labs drawn just off the main lobby. The waiting room was crowded, primarily with adults. The place specialized in treating cancer, so there was always some smoker nearby hacking loudly. Jody laughed it off and adapted easily. J and I were slower to sign on. We'd trusted the mask for months, for cover in mad dashes through the Children's lobby and in other ambiguous circumstances, and we'd gotten to Seattle without a fever. Now we were supposed to believe it was nothing more than a security blanket with ear straps? This was like telling Van Helsing the crucifix doesn't do squat against Dracula. Or telling Mom not to count on her scapular to get me through the gates.

I posted: "*The national donor center informed our docs that the donor needs to delay things by a week. We're not sure why, but are assured it's merely a postponement, and they don't need to return to the donor pool. Delays apparently are not uncommon. We'll leave the Residence Inn next week. A two-bedroom apartment has become available at the Pete Gross House, also just a short walk from the SCCA. We're told this apartment is on the fifth floor with a deck and a view of both Lake Union and the Space Needle. All in all, we consider the donor delay a minor setback, and are excited the apartment has become available.*"

The Pete Gross House was too good to be true. The building is named for the late Seattle sportscaster, a locally beloved figure, who as a Hutch patient became aware of the many who relocated from long distances for treatment. He inspired an apartment building dedicated to the patients and near enough to SCCA that some residents could walk. The five blocks included a steep climb, though, so some could not. Shuttles run several times daily between Pete Gross and the SCCA, UW Hospital and Children's. Given the ravages of treatment, some who could manage the walk one day needed the shuttle the next. Just off the lobby of the Pete Gross House is the Hutch School.

Fred Hutchinson was a major league pitcher and coach who made it to the World Series in 1961 as manager of the Cincinnati Reds. My brother Dan, who introduced me to sports writing, recalled meeting Hutch, and liking him. From Seattle originally, Hutch spent many years managing the Seattle Rainiers of the Pacific Coast League. He died of lung cancer in 1964 at age 45.

William Hutchinson, a Seattle surgeon, created a living memorial to his brother by establishing the Fred Hutchinson Cancer Research Center, which merged with Children's Hospital and UW Medical Center into the SCCA, efficiently and effectively connecting research and clinical care, in-patient and out. We felt the care of each significantly.

As I got to know the key SCCA players, my comfort with our decision to move cross-country grew. But that decision was based on drug choices and radiation doses and the specifics of approach to a disease. I'd not given much thought to the broader matter of healing philosophy. The Hutch School opened my eyes to a thoughtful, organic approach to the work of healing. J was the total focus of Jody's and my attention; she had no siblings to distract us. By comparison, most of the students of the Hutch were not patients themselves, but children or siblings of patients.

Such kids become secondary victims of their family member's disease, and in one way or another are lost, or neglected, amid the chaos and treatment. The Hutch School created a normalcy for the uprooted child, with teachers and staff who tailored education to individual needs and were gifted in the art of empathy. They knew the child's circumstance, and were unendingly patient and understanding. It cannot help healing for a patient to know their child is being neglected and to lack the energy or time to do anything about it. For an adult distracted from parenting by the demands of their own or another child's treatment, the Hutch was an extraordinary gift, and for me indicated the SCCA's comprehension of the totality of the healing process. The more comfortable J became with her tutor, Eileen, the more Jody and I could shut off our cares for blissful and brief respite. What a gift.

Moving into the Pete Gross House meant deconstructing the "safe" environment we'd created in the Residence Inn. Not wanting to trust J's health to the recirculated air of a hotel, we had brought along Hepa air purifiers and microfiber filters for the hotel and apartment vents. What they captured wasn't pretty. But we wondered what was the point when, arriving through the front door of the Pete Gross House on moving day, the building super was hard at work painting the lobby. The fumes were strong, and I had no clue about their volatile organic compounds. I zipped J through the lobby, to the elevator, and up to our sanctuary. We opened the windows.

As fumes abated and we settled in and J became more comfortable at the Pete Gross House, she could leave our apartment without us, take the elevator to the lobby and go to school by herself—without ever leaving the security of our building. This gave J a nice break from my vigilance, and a taste of independence I got comfortable with. Too comfortable. J went to a tutoring session and said she'd return on her own. When she left, I mindlessly locked the door, though I'd promised not to, and then fell asleep while reading. When she returned, the locked door and no response left J in tears in the hallway. She was hurt and upset with me. The last thing a kid in such a frightful time needs is something else to fear. She needed peace and security and confidence in her father. I had failed her, and I felt awful.

The Hutch School was not the only haven at the Pete Gross House. The balcony of our apartment provided easy access to a cooling breeze and a view sans Hooters. The elevation also brought into view the Space Needle, the Pacific Design Center, Olympic Peninsula and the downtown skyline. We could watch the seaplanes turn eastward from Puget Sound, approach from the south and begin their steep descent toward the lake, seemingly within arm's reach. From the balcony we could make out the odd shape of the Experience Music Project, a museum of rock 'n' roll designed by Frank Gehry, whose Santa Monica home had been on the route of a walk to the farmer's market that Jody and I took with some regularity before moving east. The Gehry house had chain link jutting inexplicably, incoherently, from a second-story wall. Another home he designed on the boardwalk in Venice Beach was equally inexplicable, and yet fascinating and beautiful. *And don't criticize what you can't understand.* From our perch, the colors and shapes of the EMP were something wild.

The Pete Gross House had two patios, one for sun lovers and the other for those needing shade. The former was atop the building and featured a garden of bamboo, herbs and flowers maintained with loving care. The views were 360 degrees. J and I counted cranes remaking the city. Several floors below, wings of the building formed a U-shape around the other patio. The building itself provided the shade. The view wasn't nearly as good, but too much exposure to the sun can feed graft vs. host disease, and certain meds heighten susceptibility to the sun's rays. This was architecture with SPF built right in.

Smoking was banned in all indoor and outdoor spaces except for one, a small patio off the main lobby. A smoking section made sense like chain link jutting out from the second floor. Then again, smokers in a cancer crowd are about as surprising as wizards at Hogwarts.

Jody posted: *"J needed a CAT scan this afternoon. They did a routine swab of her nasal passages last week and mold grew in the petri dish. Mold is everywhere in the environment, I'm told. No one can avoid it. But most people have the immune system to fight off mold in their system. Not J. So they needed to do a CAT scan to make sure she didn't have any in head or torso. Good news. Clean CAT scan."*

Before J became ill, I'd never donated blood with more than a vague, do-gooder's instinct. I had no real understanding of the profound and unendingly urgent need. I should have known but didn't. That changed over the course of seeing my daughter repeatedly require transfusions, and what she needed always being available. When she bled into her lung after her port surgery, and was rushed back to OR, somebody else's platelets stopped the bleeding.

I'd donated a few times when I worked at the Boston Herald, where the Red Cross would set up in the basement, but hadn't since a bout of Lyme disease rendered me ineligible. The spirochetes that cause Lyme are so hard to find, a positive test shows not the spirochetes but an increased level of antibodies in the blood—T cells in their right mind. But once antibiotics had returned the antibodies to a normal level, and the symptoms were gone, it was assumed I no longer had Lyme. That was a safe enough assumption for me, but not for the recipient of my blood. So I was banished, and didn't give it another thought until I watched, time after time, as nurses hooked J up to bags of red or platelets. I knew platelets were vital, but it was the red cells that really got to me. To watch the color return to J's face, her eyes widen, her energy leap, it was as if I had received the transfusion myself.

I thought it was worth checking if Lyme policy had changed, and it had. Symptom-free for more several years, I was eligible again. I made an appointment in the donor center just off the lobby at Boston Children's, made the trip down from Seven West, and got to work. They took a double bag that day. I got into a routine giving platelets, which last only five days, and two weeks later giving longer-lasting red cells, then repeating a couple months later.

To donate means subjecting yourself to a lengthy questionnaire probing matters of sexuality, hygiene, where you've been lately, what you did there and with whom. This is not a questionnaire edited for political correctness. If you're not prepared for the questions, they can seem blunt and personal and catch you by surprise. *Hey, I'm doing something nice, here. What's with the third degree?*

It didn't use to be that way. The donor was thanked for the kindness with virtually no questions asked. But for a generation of hemophiliacs, transfusions became a virtual death sentence, with a blood supply turned infectious. Because of those victims and others, including many aplastic anemia patients, the blood supply that sustained J through transplant was vastly safer than it had been two decades earlier. The quandary for the blood collectors is, the need is great and yet they make it difficult for the donor. But the risks are too great to do it any other way. Only recently, they've come to understand that.

J could not have either my blood or Jody's; ours collaboratively had failed her once and wouldn't get a chance at redemption. At Boston Children's, there was systemic assurance that the blood we donated wouldn't be given to J. In a system so large, the chances were low to begin with, but there was an additional check in place to make certain.

We assumed it was that way in Seattle, and when a blood drive was scheduled at the SCCA, we donated. We judged the environment safe enough for J, and she came and watched. She took some pleasure in seeing her parents get the poke for a change, but mostly she was empathic and nurse-like.

It wasn't until after we'd completed the donation that it occurred to Jody to ask whether there was a check in place to ensure our blood wouldn't be given to J. There wasn't. It seemed to be the first time they'd heard the question. Whereas the donor center at Boston Children's primarily fed that hospital, donations in Seattle fed an entire regional network. We were assured that there was virtually no chance J would receive our blood, but for parents of a child bound for transplant with a two in a million disease, there's a gap between "no chance" and "virtually no chance" you could drive an ambulance through. We could not be assured our blood would go somewhere other than the SCCA or Children's Seattle. We made a stink, and our donated blood was destroyed. I have no idea who might have needed it. I only know who couldn't have it.

We never crossed paths with Dr. Robert Hickman, though we kept hearing he'd repeatedly put off retirement and remained a presence at the SCCA. He was spoken of with reverence and pride, feelings I adopted. When someone invents something that's been implanted inside your daughter's chest to help keep her alive, you develop a certain affection.

I had developed an affection for the port-a-cath, as well. After its frightful installation, the port had an immeasurable impact on J's ability to endure her treatment, and I wasn't anxious to see it go. The port had plenty of life left in it. We weren't close to approaching the thousand-poke mark. And yet the Seattle transplant folks wanted to swap it out for the Hickman.

The port, fully implanted under the skin, posed a lower infection risk than the Hickman. Indeed, once J had healed from the installation, the port's infection risk just about disappeared. The Hickman would require much more daily attention to keep it sanitized. But we'd come to rely on the port during one-at-a-time treatment, and that period was about to end. The Hickman, with its double access lines, allowed for intravenous multitasking, and soon there would be a queue of fluids impatiently waiting their turn.

On a dummy, Nurse Pam rehearsed us on flushing and sanitizing the Hickman. Jody became the point person on that aspect of J's care, and learned that in the event of air in the Hickman, to clamp the line, put the patient on her side, and call 911. We never called 911. We did call the SCCA 24-hour line when the cap accidentally screwed off along with the flush. But there was no air in the line, no damage done, though J spent an uncomfortable night with a saline flush attached to her Hickman. She gave Jody some grief for that.

J's return to surgery tested my stoicism, but it helped to see her platelet count bumped to 97,000, twice as many as she'd possessed most of the previous seven months. J no longer minded use of the word "surgery," an attitudinal adjustment attributable to time and the comedy team of versed and propofol.

I had a last look at the port a couple of days before surgery, during an echocardiogram that showed the device rising and falling with the beating of J's heart, about the size of her fist. I was reminded of the day in summer of 1997, in an OB/Gyn's office at Beth Israel in Boston, when I first saw J's image on ultrasound. I swear, she smiled at me that day.

The EKG technician put on a video, and J glanced from the screen with her port dancing and heart pumping to one playing "The Aristocats." *Everybody wants to be a cat. Cuz a cat's the only cat who knows where it's at.* J was assured the EKG gel lathered over her accessed port was sanitary. The screen displayed two chambers and both ventricles. The EKG revealed nothing of concern with her heart. It was going strong. She was cleared for surgery.

We arrived at Seattle Children's bright and early, only to sit and wait for hours. The surgery receptionist was apologetic and explained an organ had arrived in the middle of the night by helicopter, and unlike bone marrow, the organ didn't know where to go; it needed Dr. Healey's expertise to give a child another chance. So J would have her port removed and Hickman installed by surgeon who'd been up all night on an organ transplant.

Arriving calm, apologetic, reassuring, and alert, Dr. Healey put us at ease. This was a Left Coast surgeon, maybe 6 foot 6 and with long hair tied back in a ponytail. *Dude!* He said he didn't like keeping kids waiting, especially when they hadn't had anything to eat. He said all the right things. His anesthesiologist, complete with thick Irish brogue, had us cracking up well before he dosed the versed. I thought to tell Dr. Healey about J's bleed into her lungs after the port was installed. He'd read that already but listened to me anyway. He explained that the port would be removed from the left side of her chest, the Hickman implanted on the right side. He rechecked the surgery order. It wrongly called for a bone marrow aspiration, which already had been performed, and the order was corrected. J received versed, then propofol. She was a happy kid, then fast asleep, and then she was back with us, groggily coming to, with a Hickman line exiting her bandaged chest.

The surgery was outpatient, and the deep backseat of our rental car proved a lousy place to ride after you'd been sedated and operated on. How do you secure in a shoulder harness a child who just had a catheter line installed subcutaneously from chest to neck and another device plucked from the other side? You don't. Longest, slowest four-mile drive ever. Jody sat in the back with J. My assignment was simple: Don't accelerate too quickly, brake too hard or idle too long, and get home fast. The way I drove, I'd have been honked at and one-finger-saluted all the way home in Boston.

On April Fools Day, 24 hours after surgery, J could have used another round of propofol for the removal of the surgical dressing. It was excruciating; as bad, J said, as having her nostril cauterized. But soon we were back in our new apartment, and Jody and J snuggled in to watch "Brother Bear." I passed. Ursodiol was bear enough for me.

Lucy was visiting. J performed assorted procedures on Jody, Lucy and I, using medical supplies from Marcy in Child Life. We gave thanks and enjoyed a meal prepared by Lucy, in celebration of Passover.

J posted: "*Hi people! Guess what? I have a Hickman line. That is a special line and I probably will never have to get poked again, people!*"

On the last day of Lucy's visit, she hung out with J while Jody and I attended Sunday service at the University Unitarian Church. In a sanctuary with 200 or so people, we found a row in the middle and sat down next to a woman who looked familiar to me. I nudged Jody and pointed this out, but she didn't recognize the woman and I didn't say anything until after a powerful sermon on gratitude, by a minister named Rev. Grace, when I said excuse me and asked the woman if her name was Jenny and if she was a surgical assistant to Dr. Healey. She smiled and said yes. I said we'd met just before Dr. Healey installed a Hickman line in my daughter's chest on Friday. She got this surprised look and said, *J?* She asked how J was doing, and I said fine, thanks, and then we shut up and listened to the music, and later she said she'd pass along my gratitude to Dr. Healey.

Jody posted: "*The donor has passed all the final medical clearances and we're all good to go for the transplant on Thursday, April 13th. This is great news. J will be admitted to Children's Hospital this Saturday, April 8th and will begin chemotherapy immediately on that day to prepare her body to receive the new marrow. It's hard to imagine that in 3 days we'll be beginning a 4-6 week stay in the hospital.*"

At noon the day before J would be admitted to Children's, the Hutch School organized a poetry reading for students and families. The theme was "Home." J wrote and read "A Cool Place": *Look in my house, what do you see. My parents, my cat, my guinea pig and me. Outside my house, look what's there. A big lawn, a climbing tree, and bugs everywhere. When I think of my house and the window seat, I think, Gee, this place can't be beat!*

Jody wrote and read "Home in Brookline": *Walking J to school and catching up with neighbors on the way. Talking to my friend on the phone and then passing her in the halls at work later that day. Eating a salad made from veggies that Paul grew in our own garden. Looking out the window and seeing my uncle's truck parked in his driveway, two streets over. Listening to J giggle with her piano teacher in the living room. Attending my nieces' chorus concerts with my extended family snugged into the pews at my home church.*

I didn't want to write anything, but Jody and J guilted me out of doing nothing. I googled a Mary Oliver poem, "Wild Geese," but I wimped out. Child Life specialist Marcy volunteered to read it. *Tell me about despair, yours, and I will tell you mine. Meanwhile the world goes on.*

Teachers, students and parents shared what they'd written. One woman, sporting a few weeks' growth of hair on her head, read with emotion thoughts of her home in Alaska. She was there with her husband and daughters, and I later learned she was the Hutch celebrity: Susan Butcher, Iditarod champion. Her daughters were Hutch students, but she was the one in treatment.

I was wary about attending the reading, because of the size of the crowd gathered, but Jody felt strongly that Hutch School staff and families knew to stay away if they were symptomatic. It was a hard point to argue. Being at the Hutch was almost like being on Seven West. J's lack of immune defense wasn't unique in this crowd. The diversion was welcome. Just a day earlier, standing on our balcony and seeing in the distance the Experience Music Project, with architecture said to have been inspired by a smashed Jimi Hendrix guitar, I felt like smashing something myself. *Lately things just don't seem the same.* Two days until chemo. One week to transplant.

Here's how smart they are at the SCCA. One of the first packets we received was from the Long Term Follow-Up department. Long-term follow-up is a wonderful concept to take with you to the Transplant Ward.

CHAPTER SEVEN

A Bag of Goo

In the days immediately preceding bone marrow transplantation, a countdown begins from the negative. Before hope, there must be emptiness. Before healing, depletion.

The countdown reminded me of space exploration from my childhood, the glory days of JFK and Cape Canaveral, the excitement as Cronkite or Huntley or Brinkley turned reverentially quiet and let the voice of NASA pronounce the T-minus sequence—"five, four, three, two, one ... We have liftoff." Another countdown, memorable in its own way, was to the New Year, televised from Times Square, with Dick Clark or Guy Lombardo, whoever came first. FM radio countdowns, Memorial and Labor Day bookends to summer in Southern California, inevitably arrived at "Stairway to Heaven," "Satisfaction" or, God help us, "Free Bird" at No. 1.

In transplant, countdown is not in seconds or songs, but days and doses. There is a liftoff, of sorts, or a fervent hope for one. Release from the hospital would require liftoff, and liftoff takes its time if it comes at all. Liftoff may need its own power booster.

During countdown, I stopped paying attention to counts. J's CBC would continue to indicate when more platelets or red cells were needed, but neutrophils and white cells would be negligible for weeks, in the hopeful scenario, and not worth a care. A patient who isn't neutropenic before conditioning will be during and for some time after. Dr. Robert Andrews counseled us to forget about the counts for a while, but this felt odd. ANC had for months been such a key signpost. But positive days would be well into the teens before the new marrow might begin to express its potential. In the wake of the aggressive gang tackle of conditioning, engraftment takes its time.

J's countdown began on Saturday, Day -5. No clock was ticking, unless you count the pounding in my head. We loaded up our low-backseat rental car in the Pete Gross House garage, drove to Children's Hospital and checked into the SCCA Unit at 10:15 a.m. My memory of the day is more hallucination than recollection. We met our first nurse, the effervescent Susan, and the decidedly uneffervescent Dr. Andrews, who would be the attending physician and a stabilizing daily presence through the minus and well into the plus. Dow, our physician's assistant at the SCCA outpatient clinic, had begun a month's rotation at Children's and would also be a near-daily presence. We toured the unit and moved into our room. Small but private. No chemo'd-up roommate. No Teletubby Turalura. Any wee-hour wailing in this room would be our own. On a blue Post-It, I made a note to call the Volunteer Office at Children's to arrange an in-room cut for when J's hair began falling out.

Dow smiled and told us, *Today should be boring.* If only. I'd yawn a lot, but boring was never part of the mix on Transplant. Boring requires safe assumptions, and those had vanished with the neutrophils months ago. I craved boring.

As usual, I recorded all the meds J took that morning, but then I handed over the information and responsibility for it to Susan. Checking into the hospital meant the nurses would keep track. It was a relief to let go; the responsibility would be mine again soon enough. Susan conducted assorted tests in preparation for hooking up the first bag of fludarabine, and I looked to J to measure her sense of violation and test my now-he's-looking, now-he's-not Jesus face. J clung to Jody but didn't get worked up about the beginning of this assault on her privacy, perhaps having come to accept it as a necessary evil during her time on Seven West. She was more intent on personalizing the room. We'd watched the end of *Star Wars* the night before, and she named her IV pole R2 Too. She set up her stuffed bunny Nippy in a hammock fashioned from a mask on her IV pole, as she'd done on Seven West. Susan laughed at the sight of the reclining Nippy.

In preparation for the fludarabine, Susan brought a dose of tummy-settling Zofran, a.k.a. ondancatron, pronounced like something Santa says to the reindeer in coaxing them aloft. Ondancatron did the trick, and we'd count on it often. The fludarabine dose began at 1 o'clock, and by 4 we were breathing easier. Day -5 wasn't so bad. Cyclophosphamide would arrive on Day -4, but we'd learned not to get too far ahead. A good day is a good day. The multisyllabic medicinal mix entering my daughter's body included dapsone, moxifloxacin, ceftazxiadime, acyclovir, ondancatron, fluconazole, fludarabine, ursodiol. I may be forgetting something. The nurse was keeping track. I could afford to forget.

I posted: *"Since Day Zero is the day our donor's marrow becomes J's, it is thought of in transplant circles as a second birthday. For the record, J doesn't like calling it her second birthday. "I was born once," she told me. "That's enough." Can't argue with that. I must say, J's courage is breathtaking. She knows well what's coming. And yet her spirits were remarkably high today; she even seemed kind of excited to be getting started. I asked her what to tell you. She said I should say the first day of treatment "went really really really well with no side effects. Except for a little nervousness." Easy for her to say."*

OK, let's go. J said this as Susan hooked her up to the chemo. I think she was telling Jody or me to hit the PLAY button and get the *Star Wars* DVD started, but the bag of cyclophosphamide was hanging from the pole next to a stuffed bunny in a hammock and unnervingly eager to begin its assault. So J was saying to start one dark force or another. When the chemo's about to course through your daughter's veins, the memory can yellow a bit.

The memory is clear, though, of J's anger at learning there was a poke coming. The anger was justified. She'd undergone surgery to install the Hickman, which was meant to eliminate pokes, but on the heme-onc or transplant wards, there is always another poke. The Hickman, like the port before it, kept the count remarkably low, but some procedures don't take to the Hickman, and Jody and I forgot that little fact. And so it came time to meet the bunny.

Easter Week though it was, this was the rabbit anti-thymocyte glob-ulin, or ATG, cousin to the horse serum that had failed in its task to render transplant unnecessary. The rabbit serum was being called upon for another T-cell smackdown during conditioning, but before it could be employed, J needed to be tested for an allergic reaction, which required two injections into her arm. J felt upset because we'd assured her that her myriad violations wouldn't include a poke, and because it hurt. In the context of the relentless assault of pre-transplant conditioning, a shot in the arm may seem a small thing, but pain is pain, and the anxiety has to go somewhere. Read my lips: Never say no more pokes.

Watching the chemo and rabbit serum drip into her body, I felt I might throw up myself. Such nasty fluids were coursing into her, and in such quantities. I felt physically ill.

Jody missed her home, her community, and recreated it as best she could. She plastered the walls of the hospital room with skater posters, photos of family and friends and Boston caregivers, a string of origami swans from J's Sunday school classmates, even the poster of J's favorite neighborhood pond. When the first chemo headache came, J said a few drops of water from the healing service helped some.

Jody and I traded nights spent on Transplant, and let J decide. This put her in the awkward position of choosing between parents, but she had so little say about her treatment and this gave her a welcome measure of control. It took her no time at all to decide what made her most comfortable was having her mom with her at night. She didn't want to hurt my feelings— *Is that OK, Dad? You sure?*—but she was clear with her wish. So most nights, I'd drive back to the apartment.

I updated the Carepage: *By the time I said goodnight to Jody and J a little after 7 in the evening as they settled in to watch another Star Wars movie, the Day -3 side effects had been minimal. Indeed, after a bag of red cells in midafternoon, J was all ramped up and spent an hour pedaling around the corridors of the SCCA transplant unit (calm down—she wore a helmet and there were more than two wheels involved). J paused only to goof around with a couple of clowns from the Big Apple Circus. One of them, Dr. Hamsterfuzz, cracked us up as he rode the bike into walls, and fell over repeatedly. The other, Dr. Le Fou, played the squeeze box, challenged me to a skipping race, and whizzopped a rather unpleasant amount. If you lack knowledge of what whizzopping is, it cracks kids up, offends adults, and serves as sport for Roald Dahl's giants. I'll explain no more. After that, J returned to her room and promptly fell asleep. She spiked a relatively low fever, but it came and went. Don't count on all the coming days being this good, but it's okay by me if they are.*

I also read. I sipped scotch. I took some big sips. And I noticed a small group of people socializing off the Pete Gross House lobby, including two sisters from Florida, one in town for treatment, the other for support. They were from the Dominican Republic originally. The woman in treatment, for recurrent aplastic anemia, longed for her children back home. I'd met them in the lobby, then saw them out on the smoking patio, and went out to say hi. The patient asked to hear more about J. People with aplastic anemia are a minority among the cancer horde, so it's good to compare notes. She'd developed aplastic anemia years earlier, got it under control with immunosuppressants, then the counts sank again and she went to Seattle for a transplant. They'd stepped out on the patio to socialize and smoke. They wore sweats and looked to be just back from a workout. They told me about the gym at the top of the hill where SCCA patients had privileges. She offered a cigarette and asked about J's donor.

Among many Pete Gross House residents, smoking was not viewed sympathetically. Sitting on the patio guaranteed to provoke looks. Oddly, the smokers also inspired a certain jealousy. The Pete Gross House could be a lonely place, and the smoking patio was the most social spot around. There was camaraderie and group therapy to be had, if you could get over that business about carcinogens.

The patio gathering changed depending who was outpatient and who was in, whose GVHD was acting up, who'd gone home or never would. A guy from Alabama made his living cleaning airplane engines and figured that's where the cancer came from. He'd sucked in, or soaked in, a lot of benzene getting those engines clean. His transplant seemed to be going well till that day he showed up in the smoking area with a purple face and hunched over like he'd skipped forty years overnight. A conversation about Graft vs. Host Disease made me edgy. A guy from Southern California, whose wife had been referred by City of Hope to Seattle for her recurrent cancer, chewed on a stinky stogie and talked up Jesus. Wally from Reno had a military flattop that made him look like Whitey Herzog, or maybe a humbler version of Jack Nicholson in *A Few Good Men. You can't handle the truth!* Alone at night, with Jody and J on the Transplant Ward, I valued the company, the therapy, the empathy, and the occasional smoke I bummed.

Wally mostly listened, or drifted, sighed on occasion. But one night Wally got to talking about how his wife's cancer weighed on him. She didn't have a donor yet, and soon they'd return home and wait till one turned up. He opened up about how hard it was to watch his wife's body fall apart and not have the power to do anything about it. It clearly was a big deal for him to open up this way to strangers, and he wanted us to know how big a deal. He told us about being an officer in the Navy and undergoing prisoner-of-war training—learning to keep secrets no matter what the enemy does to you. This was harder, he said. He talked about being on a nuclear sub with the power to unleash a weapon. At least he had a little control then, he said.

It didn't seem like he was trying to impress us with his finger-on-the-trigger story, but instead giving a context for how out of his control his wife's health was, and how fearful that made him. Stogie Man quoted a Psalm and talked up Jesus some more. I shared something ineloquent about how lacking control sucks. It does suck, but you'd like to say something a little more helpful. Because of Stogie Man, I recalled something said about the ubiquitous WWJD bracelets and bumper stickers. I had read Garry Wills' *Why I'm a Catholic* in search of a better grasp of why I wasn't, why I'd abandoned that aspect of my blood line. Of the question *What would Jesus do?*, Wills wrote: *That is not a question his disciples ask in the Gospels. They never knew what Jesus was going to do next.* I didn't share the thought. Wally didn't need my truisms or my doubts. I did share that I believed every Pete Gross House resident had a unique but somehow shared perspective on loss of control. If nothing else, the conversation left Wally feeling he wasn't alone, and he thanked us for that. Losing control is hard. Alone and out of control is worse.

Even for its practitioners, perhaps especially for the practitioners, bone marrow transplant possesses as much disillusionment as hope. Transplant is a desperate measure and is not attempted unless the patient's life is at serious risk and alternatives are lacking or lousy. Dr. Jerome Groopman has written compellingly of the torture a transplant doctor feels when engraftment fails. He nearly abandoned the practice himself, not for the loss of hope, but because failure can be so brutal. In providing my family a clear view of possibilities ahead of us, the SCCA shared with us the full range of patient reactions—the gratitude, the despair, the incredible joy, agony and ambiguous in-between. The bliss and the blisters.

J was being treated with medicines born as weapons of mass destruction. Survivors of the atomic bombs that devastated Hiroshima and Nagasaki suddenly lost their immune systems. The radiation wiped out bone marrow, leaving victims without the platelets to stop bleeding or the white cells to fight infection. But what if there were new marrow for them? For scientists then investigating a cure for leukemia and frustrated by a recipient's rejection of new marrow, the idea of using radiation to wipe out the leukemia and defender cells was compelling.

Groopman wrote: *The technology of marrow transplantation was conceived mainly in a dog kennel in Cooperstown, New York, during the nineteen-fifties. A young Harvard-trained physician, E. Donnall Thomas, had retreated to a hospital there to work on a research problem that had eluded a generation of blood specialists. Although red blood cells could be successfully transfused from a compatible donor to a needy recipient, marrow cells could not: the body would identify them as foreign invaders and destroy them.*

Thomas wasn't the only scientist working on marrow transplantation, Groopman wrote, *but he may have been the most persistent.*

Early transplants only worked with the marrow of perfectly matched siblings. Typing for the human leukocyte antigen, or HLA, wasn't understood. Successful transplants involving siblings not identically matched simply did not occur. So bleak were results that even Thomas got out of the business, except for transplants between identical twins. By 1967, Thomas had brought his research to the University of Washington and Fred Hutchinson Cancer Center. With his Cooperstown dogs, he had figured some of the necessities of successful transplant. He found genetic markers on white blood cells, by which he could match donor and recipient. Coming to understand this "histocompatability," Thomas observed successful engraftment among littermates in his kennel. Others didn't understand; he was harshly criticized by scientists of stature. But he persisted, and formed a team dedicated to care for the transplant patients in this emergence of hope where there had been none.

As our countdown progressed, tension grew. J could smell food a mile away, and none of it smelled good. Fevers came with the ATG. A vein in her neck pulsed rapidly, near where the port had once found its source. Having watched her heart at work during the echo, I spun it as sign of a healthy organ engaged in moving blood to combat fever. J took note of a hummingbird hovering outside our window, and pointed it out to me.

On Day -2, and for the third consecutive day, J received both chemos and the rabbit serum. All were delivered through the dual lumens of the Hickman line, and when I took her for a shower her chest looked like an aerial view of the 405 at L.A. International. At one point, there were six different fluids either flowing into her or hooked up and waiting their turn. Only J knows what it really felt like. I can only imagine. I'd rather not.

The good news was, chemo conditioning had ended. But radiation was on deck.

We'd moved cross-country to reduce the total body irradiation, or TBI, that J would receive, and we could have avoided it entirely, though that never seemed reasonable. Some radiation was necessary, we'd been convinced. It became a virtual mantra: *200 sonogray is the right amount.* But receiving even a "little" of something your parents have moved cross-country to avoid is frightening, and J was pretty worked up on Day -1. There was no facility for TBI at Children's Hospital, and so a "cabulance" was arranged to deliver us the mile or so to UW Hospital, and in other circumstances a cabulance ride might have been a hoot. Weak and battered by the chemo "flu," J was in no condition for a road trip, and wouldn't be allowed off the ward for any other purpose, but this trip wasn't optional. It was the last stop before transplant.

The UW Hospital lobby and corridors bustled with patients and staff and other reminders of our vulnerability. J wore a mask, and we raced to our destination and a private corner and got out the Purell. We checked in and waited in a small seating area. The wait seemed long, but everything was magnified that day. Once in the TBI room, J's anxiety was high, my nervous energy soothed no one, and the girls banished me to the waiting area. Jody did her best to calm J, her best only marginally better than mine. For so long chemo provided J's greatest fear, but she'd gotten through that. Now radiation loomed like a showdown with Voldemort, and J's spirit felt as sapped as her immune system. She found the seat cold and uncomfortable, they let her wear nothing but a thin robe, and she had a bloody nose that wouldn't quit. J amazed me so often with her courage, but she found no calm this day, and TBI dragged on painfully.

But then it was done. Conditioning was done. Hail a cabulance, we're ready to receive.

Back in our room at Children's, J felt nervous, hungry, beat up, and eager for something good to happen. She challenged me to convince her why transplant was such a good thing. *Tell me five good things about what has happened so far.* She demanded an answer, and I didn't have one.

But tomorrow was another day. Day Zero. More than simply benefitting from years of courageous research, we were in the midst of it. Research means *to look again.* The process doesn't stop. There's no end to what isn't known. With bone marrow transplant, everything can go right until one moment it doesn't. Success is measured in mortality rates, and doesn't require all that many years survived. The practice of medicine is about the individual and the journey at least as much as it's about knowledge of health and disease.

It used to bug me to read news of a scientific study that turned on its head what had been understood the day before. *Why can't they just get it right once and for all?* But science and science journalism sometimes amount to a riff on the Woody Allen routine in *Sleeper*, where hot fudge sundaes are the future's new health food and the only thing you can count on is that the abandoned VW Beetle will start. If you think you know, you don't. J's disease was idiopathic, meaning the doctors knew when to admit defeat, in Round 1, and change the subject from cause to cure.

What we did know: We were benefitting from farsighted research. It's what brought us to Seattle. If your disease is rare, you can't expect every doctor to understand it, really understand it, to have dealt with it over and over until patterns and clarity emerged, and if you're lucky enough to find a doctor who understands yours and what can and should be done, it is a blessing indeed. On SCCA Transplant, aplastic anemia was not an orphan on the cancer ward but a specialized problem to solve by people who made it seem not so rare. Indeed, the transplant docs found cause for encouragement in the very diagnosis, and told us. Transplant for aplastic anemia can go remarkably well. The doctors liked the odds.

J's conditioning protocol was a work in progress, pioneered by Seattle, and part of a study sponsored by the National Institutes for Health, the National Heart, Lung and Blood Institute and the National Cancer Institute. Participants nationwide would feed their information to the Center for International Blood and Marrow Transplant Research in a collaborative effort that promised to produce persuasive numbers and make aplastic anemia less of an orphan.

Earlier aplastic anemia-specific studies had resulted in the determination to continue to employ radiation in the conditioning process but at a minimal one-time dose of 200 sonogray. This is what had brought us to Seattle. I recall the words from a Joachim Deeg-led study from 2001: *Earlier trials showed evidence that patients with aplastic anemia have a poor tolerance for high-dosage TBI.* Medical studies can be incomprehensible, but this sentence could not have been clearer, and it captured what I came to believe: that Seattle had a greater understanding of the peculiarities and tendencies of aplastic anemia.

Reading the document setting out specifics of the study J would participate in is an emotional minefield, a glossary of fears past: mortality, morbidity, organ failure, graft failure, acute GVHD, opportunistic infection, chronic GVHD, early death. After the transplant, chemotherapy would conclude with methotrexate, in four doses over 11 days, and each time the nurse would don a disposable gown, gloves, and mask when handling it. Convincing a child she's doing great is a challenge when even the nurses are giving her the lead-suit treatment.

The cocktail of chemos made J feel lousy for days—like a bad case of the flu, as her doctors had predicted—and we anticipated mouth sores, sore throats and no appetite for some time to come. We began a hair watch, and were encouraged that the chemos had no immediate effect. *Don't get your hopes up.* For the headache and assorted other symptoms, a med smorgy was delivered.

J was recruited for multiple secondary studies, and we agreed in advance to participate in several, some for J's own good, others to give back to a system we were benefitting from. If it didn't require a poke or additional procedure, we were for it. How could we not help in any way we could? But that grateful and generous spirit got lost in J's days of chemo-induced misery, as we learned to vigilantly protect what privacy she had left, and to chase off unnecessary visitors. We backed out of much that we'd agreed to. Researchers are used to this, but it doesn't make their work easier or speed the advance of science.

A supercross rider from Team Yamaha came to sign autographs and give out Yamaha T-shirts. He was a celebrity, even had his own action figure, and celebrity can lift spirits on Transplant. I answered the knock at the door and checked with J to see if she was interested. She declined, but received a stuffed bear in a Yamaha shirt anyway. She recognized the brand name on her new bear's T-shirt but was confused by its association with motorcycle racing. *I thought Yamaha made pianos.*

I posted: *"It's past 7 on Thursday evening, and we're still awaiting the arrival of the donor marrow. Word that it was coming last night, and even that it had arrived in Seattle, was in error. It's not a big deal for the three of us. Kinda comical, in fact. We now anticipate J's transplant to begin around midnight tonight. Stay tuned."*

The marrow wasn't really late. April 13 had been the scheduled Day Zero, but then somehow lines were crossed, and Dr. Andrews heard it was en route on Day -1. In fact, it hadn't been harvested yet. Dr. Andrews apologized, but TBI day had been toxic in all sorts of ways, and so Jody and I felt an edgy relief. Maybe we were forgiving because of the room we now found ourselves in. It was more of a suite than a hospital room, and probably could have accommodated three patient beds. But it was ours alone, with more wall space than we had cards and posters for, and a large window overlooking a new and pristine garden whose formal ribbon cutting and dedication to Bill Gates' late mom was days away. So we were forgiving. Marrow tomorrow.

We were curious, though, when the marrow would arrive, and so we asked Dr. Andrews for an ETA. He smiled. *When the nurse tells me.*

Sometimes I'd go to church just with Mom. She always wanted to get there early and sit in the first row, front and center. Nowhere to hide. There never is with God, but the front row is particularly exposed. Mom would grow distant, kneeling and bowing her head and entering into silent prayer as she prepared for the mass to begin. A veil obscured her face. She encouraged me to mimic her, bow my head and try to get God's ear, but Mom's disappearance into some distant place came to feel odd, embarrassing, and beyond my ability to tag along. When Mom went quiet, I'd get fidgety, and if nothing else caught my eye I'd play with the brass clip on the pew, which when you let it go just right, in an otherwise silent church, made a pop that could raise the dead. That's just a saying.

Once mass began, Mom's silent prayer gave way to loud recitation as she emphatically participated in the responsories and song, as if she thought God was hard of hearing, which in fact I found him to be, but that's another story. Mom could tolerate some of my daydreaming at church, but not during the consecration. When the priest recited the prayers to transform the sacramental water, wine, and wafer into the blood and body of Jesus, she made sure I paid attention. She'd do this while attempting not to become distracted herself, so she'd keep her fervent gaze fixed on the sacrificial transformation occurring on the altar, closing her eyes, and tilting her head down when the *I am not worthy* part arrived, and still somehow reaching out with her left hand to hook me and reel me in. She'd gesture with her head to direct my attention where it ought to be. I tried to join her in her distant and mystical place, flailing fervently. God help me, I tried.

I cannot say I found that place eight months after Mom's death, but since letting go of the blood line that was my maternal spiritual inheritance, transplant night was the closest I'd come. Catholicism was the faith of both parents, but Mom took it to an extreme, and it was her faith— religion as dark obsession—that I quit. What I didn't leave behind was a fascination with the ancient and undying human need for God's love, and for a path forward. The space once held by the celestial and bearded male God of statuary and church art was occupied now as much by mystical curiosity as any real presence, with more interest in the wonder than the answer. Maybe this was the easy way out, the coward's route. What one believes carries such extraordinary power, and I've inherited a passion for the transcendent, but if I believe in anything fully now it's ambiguity. The existence of ambiguity gives me faith in God's sense of humor. I don't know the punch line, but I'm pretty sure I'm involved in the joke.

These days, whenever my faith is tempted to get specific, the specificity returns to dust and is gone in the next gust. And yet when Left Coast Brooke came into our room holding the bag of stem cells, with eyes open I saw a chalice raised, a miracle newly harvested and in progress, contained and transported cross-country on ice. Special delivery. I could almost smell the incense. I didn't bow my head, but I was filled with awe and blinked back tears.

J finished watching *Madagascar,* complete with Louis Armstrong singing "What a Wonderful World," and drifted toward dreamland. The 277ml bag of stem cells arrived on the ward around 10:55 p.m. in a beer cooler, white on the sides, red flip lid, tan handle. You've seen one just like it at the beach or the park. The delivery guy came and went fairly quickly. An ID tag dangled from his neck. Middle thirties, I'd guess, brown T-shirt wet from sweat or rain, dark hooded sweatshirt, head shaved and/or bald from causes unrelated to chemo, I'm guessing. He could've been delivering pizza. I didn't think to tip him.

It took a half-hour or so for the nurses to check the paperwork, make certain all the details were right—that this was, in fact, the marrow intended for J. There were no other transplants on the ward that night, but still. Jen, one of J's favorites, was the charge nurse for the night, and she posed holding the bag. Along with J's name and ID number, the label read:

HEMATOPOIETIC PROGENITOR CELLS

MARROW (HPC-M)

ALLOGENEIC

The marrow posed for more photos. By 11:30, Left Coast Brooke connected it to J. The IV pole was a crowded place. The marrow hung beside two bags of fluid, a meter, and a couple of stuffed critters in hammocks. A smaller label read:

COLLECTION DATE/TIME: 4/13/06   0614.

EXPIRATION DATE/TIME: 4/15/06 0614.

Time is of the essence.

Made drowsy by the time and a dose of benadryl, J fell fast asleep by 11:40, her head resting on her blue fish pillow Float. I stared, breathed deeply, and watched the bag, the catheter, and the deep red fluid drawn by gravity toward the Hickman and on into J's chest, where I'd been told it knew where to go and what to do. I shuddered and felt as if something ineffable entered my own body, like a reversal of the sensation the day I felt the air suddenly sucked from me and I shook and sobbed uncontrollably as the lid dropped on my father's coffin. Some stranger's marrow entered my daughter and was about to take up residence—a long residence, I hoped and even prayed for, though don't ask me to what or to whom. I couldn't have been more present in that room, and yet I'd landed in a distant and mystical place as well, existing at once in first and third person, a magical realm maybe Gabriel Garcia Marquez could explain, and I experienced a clarity that may never come again, a profound awareness of a some stranger's gift of another chance for my daughter, and I had no chance of comprehending why this was happening.

As with my desire to understand what caused J's illness, I just had to let go, accept it, and stare in wonder. J's brains, bones and tissue had my DNA, and will forever, but her blood and her hope came from someone I'd not met, a total stranger, some anonymous human being, and I had a front-row seat for this mystical transformation. J became connected to a blood line that had nothing to do with me, nothing to do with Jody, and everything to do with being alive. If God doesn't exist in that transaction, God doesn't exist.

Jody had bought a bottle of red wine to celebrate—Rodney Strong, same as we'd poured at our wedding reception. We opened it, toasted and hoped. A schoolmarm of a nurse later let us know this was not okay, that wine didn't belong on the transplant ward. *We don't need no stinking metaphors!* We could accept that the rule on some level was appropriate, and so I poured the California Cabernet down the drain, ran the water after it, and left alone what the two became. Just water and wine, down the drain.

Before falling asleep, J became fed up with Jody and me making a fuss about the arrival of the marrow. We giggled nervously, marveled, and posed holding the bag while Left Coast Brooke snapped our picture. J wondered aloud what was the big deal? *It's just a bag of goo!*

We had to wait till she was asleep to take her picture with the bag. In it, the bag hangs to J's left, and she's watched over by an autographed poster of Belbin & Agosto, the ice skating pair and among J's new Olympic heroes. She'd told Lucy how much she'd enjoyed the Olympic figure skating. You don't tell such things to Lucy expecting a simple *That's nice, honey,* and nothing more. Lucy got on the phone, of course, talked to a friend with NBC Sports connections, and before the Zamboni had smoothed the ice, there was Lucy in Seattle with a sleeve of autographed photos. Johnny Weir, Sasha Cohen, Irina Slutskaya, notable among many others. The night the new marrow arrived and took residence, the saints watching over my sleeping daughter wore skates. The guardian angels, well, they wore what nurses wear, and they worked until their shift was done.

The next morning, Jody posted: *"J has been sleeping, sleeping, sleeping for the whole day. I'm glad her body is getting a break because she was up all last night feeling very sick. But I miss her sweet smile and energy. Last night was such a roller coaster."*

J loves her Aunt Wrapping Paper and especially loves visiting her house in Santa Rosa, California. Aunt WP keeps cockatiels and parakeets, and arranged a bathroom for the birds to leave their cages and chirp and squawk and flutter and sit on J's shoulder while nibbling on her cheek. J hung out in there for hours. A few months after our August 2005 visit, with J no longer possessing a functioning immune system and isolated from animals of any sort, Aunt WP informed me one of her birds had died, and she worried there might be a connection to J's illness. *West Nile?*

We had all kinds of theories about the possible cause, but no answer to what it was; that will never change. I told my sister her late bird was an unlikely culprit, and that anyway the doctors had ruled out what they could, stopped looking for a cause, and moved on to focus exclusively on a solution.

That we pursued our solution in Seattle meant good news for Wrapping Paper. Flights from San Francisco or Oakland are less of an ordeal to Seattle than to Boston, making her visits easier. When I lived in Southern California, our visits were more frequent. I knew her sons well growing up, was godfather to one, confirmation sponsor to the other, though not before Mary Jo and I discussed why I couldn't make certain Catholic promises in good conscience. She and I have had so many conversations of that sort, through her divorce and mine, and through her years caring for our parents.

Aunt WP collects stuff. Much of it she individually wraps, gathers into large boxes and ships to J for one occasion or another. The potential occasions were made limitless by J's illness. Thus was born my sister's nickname. Of course, she also collects stuff and doesn't ship it, and so her home is full of tchotchkes and photos and refrigerator magnets and memories and assorted message cards meant to get one through the day. Henry Miller on being alive. Churchill: *If you're going through hell, keep going.* There's Lao Tze, Dylan, and Mother Teresa, though I forget what they said. One card offers tips for how to teach and how not to. There's a vintage Howdy Doody trivia poster. Garfield in a nightcap saying *I'll rise but I won't shine.* I get crazy with the clutter, but J scowls at me if I mention it, and each piece means something special to Aunt WP. Truth is, I'd miss them if they were gone, except maybe that late seventies photo of me and my brothers at Steve's wedding, looking like album art from Air Supply.

My personal favorite is an old comic clipped from a daily newspaper. It's a one-panel image of three game-show contestants standing at individual podiums. Two of them have $0 showing on their tally boards. The third contestant, in flowing white hair, beard and robe, has thousands of dollars in winnings, and holds a board displaying his answer: *What is the Pythagorean theorem?* The caption: *God, kicking some serious butt on Jeopardy.*

Aunt WP's stuff collection includes a small library devoted to Mother Teresa, and she takes many of the late nun's principles to heart whether caring for an elderly parent or teaching trombone to a child, inevitably poor and Hispanic in an underfunded school that has seen families of means flee for a private education. Like Mother Teresa, Aunt Wrapping

Paper takes better care of other people than of herself, and she's forever striving to correct that. She speaks in multidirectional staccato bursts. She's never said anything so concise it could fit on one of her refrigerator magnets. She loves to laugh. I could tell the same story a hundred times and she'd laugh just as hard in the latest retelling, though that would require an opening in her running commentary. J especially loves her aunt's stories about me as a little boy. I don't remember all that much; Aunt WP forgets nothing, and never tires of the telling. She came to spend Easter with us.

I posted: "*I'm not going to get too heavy-handed with the Easter metaphor, but I must say, J barely lifted her head off the pillow on Friday, managed a bit of playfulness out of bed on Saturday, and then, boom, she was back, bright and early Sunday morning, playing with the magic kit and the handcuffs that the Easter Bunny brought her. For the record, she's getting a bit suspicious of the Easter Bunny. And as for the handcuffs in an Easter basket, well, direct those questions to Jody. Dr. Andrews and the physician's assistant Dow Dunbar ('I like Dow,' says J) dropped by Sunday morning to find J sitting by the window offering to perform tricks. 'I think you already performed some magic,' Dr. Andrews said. 'What did you do with J?'*"

There is no medical innovation without desperation. I distrust simple truth but feel fairly safe with this one. The healing trade is supply and demand at its most urgent, which perhaps is why so many advances are born of war. Douglas Starr, a professor of science journalism, wrote compellingly of this in *Blood: An Epic History of Medicine and Commerce*. I can't imagine opening such a book before J's illness infused my consciousness and curiosity with some stranger's stem cells. I wanted to know who to thank, to better ground my gratitude and fend off my fears.

Certain characters leapt off the pages of *Blood*. Karl Landsteiner, in early 20th century Vienna, ran blood experiments, kept notes, spotted and documented trends. He was first to name blood by type, and to note how different types reacted when mixed. Understanding blood's properties, differences in type, and need for sterile procedures had begun.

Around the same time, Alexis Carrel, a visionary vascular surgeon, immigrated to Canada and then to the United States when he found his research and clinical work compromised and marginalized in his native

France. Carrel was among the scientific innovators recruited in 1906 to the research institution being created in New York by the philanthropist John D. Rockefeller—an almost idyllic place for great minds to pursue their research. Carrel brought his study of blood vessel engraftment using cats and dogs.

In the predawn hours of a Sunday in March 1908, Carrel was approached at his home by Dr. Adrian Lambert and his two surgeon brothers. Lambert's infant daughter could not stop bleeding from the nose and mouth. He knew of Carrel's work and asked him in desperation to save his daughter. Carrel had no surgical license but was convinced to disregard ethical and legal questions, and to do what he could to save a child's life. He strapped the infant to an ironing board atop the dining-room table, bound the father's wrist to her leg, and tried to connect an artery of Lambert's to a tiny vessel in the baby. "He failed several times, ripping through the walls of the tissue-like vein, before finally connecting them," Starr wrote.

The blood flowed from father to daughter to no immediate effect. Then an uncle saw "a little pink tinge at the top of one of the ears," the lips went from blue to red, the child from ghostly white to baby pink, and then the infant cried. "You'd better turn it off or the baby will bust," an uncle said. Carrel clamped off the blood vessels and tied them. The baby survived, and circulation in the father's hand was restored.

I'm jealous of the father. My blood was of no use to J. Then again, I wouldn't change eras. I wouldn't swap J's care in the early 21st century for the Lambert child's in the early 20th. We had options, and even with our mystery disease we were beneficiaries of remarkable understanding and advanced practice born of a century of imaginative, desperation-driven work. We'd made it to transplant after about eighty successful blood transfusions, all from strangers.

The Lambert mother subsequently wrote a letter to Rockefeller, in the persona of her baby, expressing gratitude for having made a place for Carrel to pursue his life-saving art. Carrel won a Nobel Prize in 1912. I think his dogs and cats deserve a share in the glory, along with the embroiderer from Lyon, France who taught him to stitch.

On the transfusion timeline, Carrel's work marked a breakthrough. There'd been attempts at human healing using calf's blood going back to the 1600s, and though essentially banned as quackery for more than a century, curiosity persisted about the properties and power of human blood until the first human to human transfusion in 1818. James Blundell, a London obstetrician, transfused ten patients over a decade, and half survived, according to Starr.

Whether or not they knew it, the Lamberts owed a debt to the social struggle with modernism, and another child's cure. Before Carrel left France for North America, a young patient survived a bacterial abdominal infection that Carrel had assumed would kill her. Carrel, a spiritual man, had accompanied the girl to Lourdes, long considered miraculously curative among those Catholics with a Marian devotion—Catholics such as my mother, who was rarely without Lourdes water and borderline bereft when lacking.

Carrel encouraged the girl's hospitalization, but instead she was doused with holy water and prayer. The girl's symptoms inexplicably abated, Starr wrote, and Carrel "described what he saw in a report to the Lyon medical community, and candidly answered questions from the press." He was scorned by his medical fellows for even considering a mystical component in cure, and by the church for crediting anything but.

A victim of intolerance for ambiguity, Carrel didn't wait for a miracle to transform his reputation in his native country. He left for North America, carrying with him an enduring bitterness toward what Starr described as "rigidity and closed-mindedness" in his homeland. He would attend Mary Robinson Lambert's 21st birthday. A social worker with the Neurological Institute in New York, she was 34 when she died of a brain hemorrhage.

On Transplant, while I rooted for a stranger's bone marrow to make itself at home inside my daughter, I assisted her in the surgical removal of Aunt Wrapping Paper's vocal cords. It was another pretend attempt at silencing someone none of us want silenced. But Aunt WP speaks the language of whiplash, and not even advanced GPS could follow her trip from opening thought to closing punctuation. Performing play surgery seemed to give J some sense of control over what was transpiring in her own real world. Aunt WP understood this and willingly played along, even at the possible loss of her own loquaciousness.

J did yoga with Linda, the occupational therapist, teaching as much as she learned. We got word that Marcy's internship in Child Life was ending. We missed her already. J's mouth was showing little of the expected side effects of chemo, though the dentist was concerned about her cracked lips. Open wounds, even little ones, aren't taken lightly on Transplant. The dentist suggested we use lanolin at night. J hated it. Dr. Andrews checked in, saw nothing worrisome, and said methotrexate's downside should have shown its ugly face by now. There'd been blood in J's eye, but Dr. Andrews said it was draining downward and would soon disappear. He said he wasn't concerned, so neither was I. I gave the Jesus eyes a rest.

Back at the Pete Gross House, an email said Amelia Quinn's Carepage had been updated. I logged in to read, in her mother's words, that Amelia had died at Saturday on Seven West. She was going to be a doctor. She'd have begun med school in the fall. She needed a transplant, and no donor had been found. J had a few hundred potential matches, and Emily had none.

I had passed her in the hall, smiled and said hi, but never got to know her. But Seven West and the Carepages formed a unique community. I posted a Carepage update from Seattle about the percolating promise of J's new marrow to, among others, an extended community in mourning. I chose my words with care.

Suggestion: Never tell a parent whose child has just died that he or she has gone to a better place. You don't know that, and though it might make you feel better, it doesn't help. If you lack for something helpful to say, this makes you pretty much like everyone else, so offer your condolences and leave it at that. Be present and empathic with the living and don't presume to know the forwarding address of the newly dead. You don't know what you think you know.

Mom would disagree with me, but she's gone. To a better place, perhaps, where no one's snapping the brass clip.

Chapter Eight

Left Coast Brooke & Other Forces of Nature

J hates when I joke about Harry Potter. She breathes a certain drag-on fire if I dare to criticize the story, as when I made a point about not liking the way J.K. Rowling factors the overweight condition of Uncle Vernon and Cousin Dudley into what makes the family on Privet Drive so detestable. I admit it; I have a target's sensitivity to fat jokes. Harry's relatives are a beastly lot, but using obesity as a measure of the beastliness feels mean.

Such talk is sacrilege to J, like I'd belittled Mother Teresa to Aunt Wrapping Paper, Freud to Jody. Even to me, such criticism feels ungrateful, because I do love Harry Potter and his magical story, and feel a debt to their creator. J repeatedly read the books, viewed the DVDs and especially listened to the shape-shifting Jim Dale bring the characters to life on CD. The wizards, Weasleys, werewolves and Whomping Willows populated a welcome alternate universe during the journey through her own personal Azkaban. So maybe I should swig a little Polyjuice Potion and get over it.

Anxiety built toward release of the seventh and final book, with so many young and old nervously wondering—*Will Harry die?* Not knowing was excruciating.

You don't need more than the title of the opening chapter—*The Boy Who Lived*—to understand the tale to be loaded for a child comprehending mortality. Indestructible, that Harry. And so brave he speaks aloud the name of He Who Must Not Be Named. *Voldemort!* There, I said it. For a while, surgery needed a euphemism with J. Then, poof!, surgery became surgery.

With his wiles and his wand, Harry made facing danger an adventure by transcending fear. OK, I'm weakening. The Dursleys can be fat.

In her bed on the transplant ward, J had control not of a wand but of a handheld device that allowed her certain levitation powers. She could

151

make her bed elevate and descend at her whim. She could make it rise quite high, enough that climbing off required a drop, much less than from a top bunk but more than, say, 250,000 platelets stacked. This made some nurses merely nervous but prompted others to insist she lower the bed. Lacking their own wand to make platelets cook more quickly, the nurses wished for any fall to begin closer to the floor.

J could manipulate the bed into assorted positions. Tethered to the IV pole because she'd consumed nothing but bagged lipids through the Hickman, she needed a position that stayed comfortable, which was the only position she couldn't achieve. I'd have spoken a curse to give the bed that quality—*Horizonto Relaxomicus!*—but that's just the sort of sacrilege that'd make J go Snape on me. Harry Potter demanded to be taken seriously. I was slower than a stem cell understanding this.

SCCA staff worked tirelessly to fill patients' days with more than bags of fluid, cups of pills, and *Let's have a look* poke-abouts. There were tutors, physical therapists, music therapists, Child Life specialists, honking and farting clowns, the odd celebrity cyclist and a parade of volunteers stopping by to see if they might be the one to make a difference in a bleak existence. J had parents and visiting family and friends, nurses and doctors, and generally preferred her peace, quiet and headphones to an unexpected visit from a kind human she didn't really know. We said thanks, but passed.

Even when J was feeling lousy, though, she never said no to Julie or Marcy from Child Life. They could change an entire day's mood with a five-minute visit. *Must you go already?* Eileen the tutor had that gift, as well, but was handicapped by her determined focus on math facts. Linda the physical therapist scored points by helping J make a cast for stuffed Monk Monk and delivering a four-wheel pedal vehicle. It was the Hummer of go-karts, and the fact we could park it in our room is an indication of our space.

J loved that cart. Seeing it parked there motivated her to eat and drink more regularly, so she could get unplugged from the IV more frequently. Linda and the others were specialists in the healing aspect of spirit, gifted at infusing joy and optimism. That cart pulled quite a load.

Volunteers had less success. J developed a look that said wordlessly but clearly, *Dad, don't even ask, just politely tell them to leave.* Many knocked, but few were chosen. Then came Solomon.

A middle-aged man, soft-spoken and engaging, Solomon didn't push it when J declined his initial offer to come in and play for a while, but before leaving he ascertained her interest in Harry Potter and in Legos, and when he returned days later, he carried a Lego hockey player and a paperback *Chamber of Secrets.* J thought the hockey player a curious choice but invited Solomon in to construct it with her.

J became nearly as absorbed by Lego as by Harry Potter, and Jody went online to find a hybrid—a Lego set from *Goblet of Fire.* Say what you will about importing a play graveyard onto a transplant ward. J lowered her bed and dove right in, snapping the scene together, then collaborating with her mom on a short film, which J wrote, narrated and chose a soundtrack for. It was a dark and stormy tale.

Jody posted: *"All the nurses and doctors tell us how amazed they are that J is doing so well. I don't want to get ahead of ourselves but we are feeling really lucky. Most kids by this time are getting lots of mouth sores and throat sores (late effects of the chemo). But J is doing so well she's even begun nibbling a bit, though she's still on liquid IV nutrition."*

J was getting another chance, and I was going to seed. My job, as I saw it, was to do what I could to give her a fighting chance, and one key way to do that was to mirror hope, not fear, and in many ways I was doing a damned good job of it. But there was this physical reality: an inescapable mirror of depression and sloth.

My daughter was having time added to her life and I was subtracting from my own. People cut you a lot of slack when your daughter has a life-threatening illness, so nobody said anything, but it pretty much went without saying. My pants were tight, and they were my fat pants to begin with. My lower back ached from weakness in my gut. I got winded going up stairs. I couldn't remember breaking a sweat. My way of letting off steam involved scotch and bummed cigarettes. I told Jody I wanted to look into the gym near the Pete Gross House that the Dominican sisters told me about. We both joined.

The gym was in a UW medical building built at elevation into what, across the monolithic Interstate 5, becomes Capitol Hill. Rows of machines faced a westerly view of the Space Needle, Puget Sound, the Olympic Peninsula, and a parade of descending seaplanes. Staff asked regularly about my daughter.

The gym became invaluable to Jody and I separately, and we'd work out together when the stars aligned, but it was only convenient to the Pete Gross House. While staying at Children's Hospital, we'd hike or bike along Burke-Gilman Trail or through Lindenhurst, with its stunning Lake Washington views.

Near the hospital, trails at UW's Center for Urban Horticulture meandered with the curves of Lake Washington, whose shoreline was alive with turtles sunning on driftwood, great blue heron spearing food along the banks among an ornithologist's dream gathering of birds, and this odd critter that I thought was a beaver until Jody pointed out the tail, which was nothing like the beaver's paddle and more like a rat.

I came upon these peculiar critters on successive walks, and assumed them to be muskrats until one day I heard a story about them on NPR. They were nutria, and it struck me as a funny coincidence that on my breaks from neutrophil watch I should happen upon a mammal known as nutria. It's like they'd been invented for the occasion.

In fact, nutria behave much in the manner we hoped the neutrophils would—they reproduce like crazy. Also like J's new marrow, the nutria were imported. Nutria are native to South America. The word itself is Spanish for otter. They're known as swamp rats and bog bears, probably by people who've watched the voracious critters devour their beloved wetland vegetation. In that way, they're like deranged T cells.

Somebody apparently brought some to the Northwest with a scheme to use their pelts to make money, never found a market, and released them. In South America, alligators keep the numbers down. There are no alligators in Lake Washington, or any other predators other than humans with cage traps, so the beasts devour the marshland grasses and make babies. They had it pretty good, and for better or worse were thriving, a quality we hoped to see in neutrophils.

The building housing the staff of the Center for Urban Horticulture was brand new. It had been built to replace one destroyed in a 2001 fire-bombing by members of the Earth Liberation Front. The eco-terrorists went after the UW center mistakenly convinced that the scientists there were engaged in genetically altering poplar trees. The center's scientists were working with poplars, but in a more traditional study of cross-breeding the fast-growing trees as a means of giving timber companies a logging alternative to natural forest. When the bombers hit the UW center, colleagues simultaneously burned a poplar farm in Oregon. Environmental activism has strong roots in the movement to halt logging of natural forests, so it was ironic that they burned work devoted to that cause. But ideology always interferes with judgment.

Environmental extremists decry modernism generally. I grew up thinking of modernism as some fearful godless plot to destroy the world, thanks to Mom and the literature and voices she surrounded herself with, but you don't have to grow up breathing brown air and topping off your tank along the endless freeways of LA going nowhere fast to realize there's a moral in there somewhere. Mom was no tree-hugger, but she was never the same after her church embraced modernism with Vatican II.

A writer friend convinced me I needed to discover Ian McEwan. Ready for a break from Edinburgh and Detective Rebus, I bought a paperback copy of *Saturday*. The events of the novel are contained within 24 hours, and a reader isn't likely to take a single day lightly again. Or maybe that's just me and the wake-up call that was J's illness.

The protagonist of *Saturday*, Henry Perowne, is a neurosurgeon, and McEwan's descriptions of the brain and the cutting are exquisite. He wrote of Perowne's mother: "She was a woman who gave her life to housework, to the kind of daily routines of polishing, dusting, vacuuming, and tidying that were once common, and these days are only undertaken by patients with obsessive compulsive disorder." Add a phrase about spiritual devotion, and McEwan could have been writing about Mom. When a century sees cleanliness turn symptomatic, the pace of change is fearful.

Anti-modernists attack science, and science was saving the life of my anti-modernist mother's granddaughter. But I'll get off the soapbox.

Better to put my Weasley butt on an elliptical cross-trainer with a view of the forests and peaks of the Olympic Peninsula. God's country, that.

My sister was visiting, and got Jody away from the hospital for a night. In a Carepage post about waiting, she wrote: "It was nice to feel fresh air on my face at night. I miss my life in Brookline so much – my house, my neighborhood, my church, my work, my analyst, my friends and my sweet family. But I wouldn't want to be anywhere else right now."

I tried not to pass the threshold into neurosis, but that's easier said than done when you're sitting around coaxing stem cells. I got to taking fiction too seriously. It was bad enough that J.K. Rowling belittled the Dursleys for being fat, now Ian McEwan was pissing me off.

In *Saturday,* Perowne listens to Steve Earle's *El Corazon*. I have that CD. It is powerful and intelligent from start to finish. So why did Perowne have to spoil it by calling Earle the "thinking man's Bruce Springsteen."

Either on LP or CD, I have most albums from both artists, play them about equally, and nobody except Dylan more. And maybe on some level I can see the fictional cranium cutter's point. Both find poetry in the day to day and nobility in the blue collar and down-and-out. Earle is Woody Guthrie to Springsteen's John Steinbeck.

Maybe Earle's progressive eloquence, his plaintive conjuring of Emma Goldman and Malcolm X and Jesus to an America that has lost its soul, elevates him in the eyes of McEwan's surgeon. Earle hits harder than Springsteen and swings more often. Maybe the Springsteen slight bugged me because I'm still angry for the time I didn't mute my stereo fast enough after *Steve's Last Ramble,* and so heard Earle loudly proclaim to my daughter, *Let's magnetize this mother fucker,* before launching into *Galway Girl.* You almost never have to mute Springsteen.

In concert Earle mostly preaches to the choir. Not a lot of Young Republicans out there swaying and holding up lighters to *Amerika 2.0.* Springsteen reassures where Earle provokes. To paraphrase the unthinking man, Springsteen's a uniter, not a divider. But maybe that's Perowne's point, and it's the challenge inherent in Earle's lyrics that elevates him to "thinking man."

Jody and I snuck away from Transplant to the University Unitarian Church for a Sunday service. An NPR reporter and author on book tour gave an eloquent antiwar sermon using strong, blunt language and solid reporting, and there was little he said that I would disagree with, and yet here he was delivering his Bush bash to a roomful of Unitarians, where there were about as many contrary views as there were white blood cells in my daughter. I like my religion least when it feels like town meeting or an independent bookstore.

Ironically, in *Saturday,* McEwan reaches movingly across a cultural divide—like Springsteen, really. Tolerance and empathy go further than anger. Mom used to listen in the L.A. wee hours to Ray Briem, who was the thinking conservative's Rush Limbaugh, and, before sending me off to the Catholic grade school, she'd cook breakfast to some John Birch radio nut who called himself Doctor and could wedge the divide with the greatest of calm.

So maybe I'll give Earle points for thinking and make Springsteen the thoughtful man's Steve Earle. Or maybe I should stop obsessing.

Perowne was a fisherman, with a favorite spot in Scotland's western highlands. "He and Jay fished the streams and lochans around Torridon for brown trout. One wet afternoon, glancing over his shoulder while casting, Henry saw his car a hundred yards away, parked at an angle on a rise of the track, picked out in soft light against a backdrop of birch, flowering heather and thunderous black sky—the realization of an ad man's vision—and felt for the first time a gentle, swooning joy of possession."

I know the place. Jody, J and I ventured to Torridon after Jody hooked us with her obsessive guidebook research, which makes me a little crazy when we travel and I have to carry all that dead weight, but always leads us to wonderful places, places I'd not discover without her and wouldn't want to. Someday I'll just say, *Tell me where to go,* and then I'll shut up and drive. We'll wind up somewhere amazing.

We stayed in Torridon in a lodge frequented by hikers and fishers. One afternoon Jody stayed in our room and napped and J and I drove to the north side of Torridon bay. J bored of the drive, but the view was stunning, reminiscent of the waters the Durmstrang ship surfaces from in *Goblet of Fire.* At the lodge's buffet breakfast, there was granola and fresh fruit and soft cheese. Within weeks, doctors at Boston Children's would want to know if J had eaten soft cheese lately, and I'd tell them about the breakfast buffet in the Scottish Highlands and wonder, *Did this start in Torridon?* I still wonder that, but only when I have no fictional characters to argue with.

J didn't feel like hiking the day we walked on moss, muck and heather through Torridon's rhododendron forest to the waterfall and up Ben Damph. She and I sat and snacked while Jody persevered and made it to the top for what payoff I cannot recall. For most of the hike, J protested that she wasn't up to it, and she wasn't. She wasn't up to the hike, and I wasn't up to the parenting. Fuck retrospect.

Sitting in the Seattle hospital room, I read a lot. I couldn't watch the news or listen to NPR much. Images from Baghdad and descriptions of exploding backpacks in crowded markets weren't the messengers of hope any healer would prescribe.

But I couldn't help myself the day Americans marched to protest the rising anti-immigrant fervor in Washington, D.C. Traffic in Seattle was a mess, and some doctors and staff ran late as a result. I had the TV on and became emotional watching. J asked me about what all the people in the streets were up to, and I explained, as we sat in our hospital room waiting and hoping her body would tolerate some stranger's marrow and let it reignite her immune system, that these mostly Mexican immigrants and supporters were marching proclaiming their right to be here.

We talked about legal and illegal immigration, about decency and fairness, about how seldom we stop and think, before picking up the knife and fork, whose hands harvest our meal. We talked about Celia, the woman from Mexico who helped Aunt Wrapping Paper care for Mom almost daily for years after Dad's death and who was stroking Mom's hand the moment she died, and tells this powerful story, when she can keep her emotions in check, about Mom's unusual presence and awareness of her world during her last day.

J and I discussed the different meanings of tolerance, cultural and immunological, or I talked and she listened, and then she got tired of the conversation and asked if we could change the channel. Push come to shove, I land on the side of the stranger's marrow and the immigrant.

My Earle-Springsteen rant notwithstanding, *Saturday* was a remarkable book, 24 hours sanctified. But I'd had enough fiction. I read a *New York*

Times review of *Black and Blue*, setting Sandy Koufax's last season with the Dodgers against the civil rights struggle circa 1966, and bought a copy. I was a Dodger fan as a kid, and followed them casually right up till Rupert Murdoch bought the team and I confronted my limit for tolerance. I got Koufax's autograph when I was J's age, give or take. I lived maybe 10 miles from Watts; light years, really. When Watts burned, I remember some of the images on TV, but it didn't feel like my town that was in flames.

At J's age, I loved the Dodgers but had a well-oiled Brooks Robinson mitt and no clue what Frank Robinson was so angry about.

The positive side of transplant is slow and emerges in stealth. The negatives are in your face. First a strand or two, eventually clumps.

Hair loss isn't idiopathic; you know where to put the blame. Cyclophosphamide's business wasn't inside J's head, but the fluid isn't discriminating and unlike marrow doesn't know where to go. Born of war, chemo could be metaphorically traced back centuries to Culloden in Northern Scotland, where the axes and swords swung until limbs and opposition were severed, collateral damage be damned. We saw those battle grounds from the rental van a week or so before J's symptoms became obvious, but she was bored by the story and the place, and we kept driving.

Cyclophosphamide is ruthless and efficient. In J's in adulthood, perhaps it will have been rendered unnecessary and archaic and relegated to a chapter on medical history. One can hope. The speed of science is breathtaking, and so goddamn slow.

When I didn't like a food Dad thought was good for me, he'd say, *It'll put hair on your chest.* I'm not sure what he'd say about cyclophosphamide. It is infused during treatment known, with no ironic intent, as conditioning.

In the week or so after chemo, J's lovely head of hair seemed unaffected, and Jody and I fantasized that we were somehow the exception. Dr. Andrews discouraged getting our hopes up. He knew our hopes were better invested elsewhere. And over the days, J's hair lost its silkiness and was drying out. Soon it began to disengage, mat, and make patterns on her pillow.

J watched hair come off in her hand in the shower. I asked if this bothered her. *Why? It's just hair, and there must be a bazillion kids here who are bald.* I couldn't have agreed more, but I sensed that maybe her words spoke more to how she wanted to feel than how she actually felt.

The hair loss was steady, the matting pronounced. J was irritable and confused. Follicles were everywhere, on everything. Her sheets and pillow case needed frequent changing. Her shirts made her itchy, as did the knit hats that covered the evolution from bad hair day to no hair day.

We encouraged her to let us arrange for someone to come to the room and cut it all off, but she wasn't ready and we didn't force it. She couldn't say no to the chemo; if she didn't want a haircut, so be it.

The days outside were sunny and warm, and J was frustrated when Jody or I would talk about how nice it was. She complained again about the itchiness of her hats, so I took them outside to a bench near the lower Children's entrance and sat amid the trees, blooming gardens and animal sculptures, and endeavored to remove the offending hair. At first I picked strand by strand, but this was slow going and not terribly therapeutic or effective, so I advanced to rapid stroke/pluck motions. In the warm breeze, strands and small clumps floated like bubbles in the sunlight, glistening. A woman walking by couldn't help a knowing smile, a glance full of empathy or sympathy, maybe both; a kindness drive-by.

As strands escaped my grasp, J's former hair sparkled in the sunlight like raindrops in Nairn. The day I played 36 holes on those splendid North Sea links, after a dip with J in the hotel pool, I took a walk along the shore back toward the golf course. Wind was blowing hard in my face as I walked toward a sun setting beyond Wester Ross and the highlands, and from the scattered clouds it began to rain in a most unusual way. The wind was hurling the drops sideways, into my face, but I had no desire to turn from the onslaught, such was its beauty. The raindrops were backlit by the descending sun and colored by blue sky and turned to diamonds. I stood and stared until the soaking overcame the beauty, and then I turned and went back to the hotel.

The winds of Seattle were not bringing the strands of J's hair back to me and slapping my face, but taking them away, like released birthday balloons. There was something of a letting go at work in me. I took a slow, wavering breath, and exhaled deeply. The knit caps never completely gave up the hair, retaining a residual itchiness. I imagined it felt to J like a wool sweater feels to me. I don't wear wool sweaters.

As J's hair became increasingly matted and impossible to comb or brush, the subject was equally problematic. So we discussed my hair instead. Before my hair began its slow, steady and selective abandonment of my head, I liked to grow it out. I had a ponytail when Jody and I got married. I rode to the wedding with my brother in a convertible, and arrived with a certain Charlie Manson Meets Don King look. Jody said *I do* anyway.

The grayer I got and the thinner my hair became, the tail grew less like a pony and more like, well, a nutria. That's Spanish for otter.

I stubbornly resisted giving into the aging realities of my head, and still go rather long periods between cuts, but the mirror doesn't lie. J will let me know when I've gone too long. *You've got the Einstein thing going.* This is said uncritically, matter-of-factly, though by no means is a compliment in the intellectual sense. When it comes to hair, admitting defeat isn't in the McLean blood. We'll see how donor blood feels.

A woman from a swishy local salon came to Seattle Children's weekly for chemo cleanup. We made sure she knew mine might be the only head shorn. J had some creative ideas for my new look, and opted for a mohawk. I was agreeable, but warned J that if I felt too goofy, it was coming off. I agreed to have it colored—again, with the stipulation. J wanted hot pink. I balked. She came back with orange. She was getting warmer. We decided on blue.

Left Coast Brooke suggested I try costume shops. The next morning, I awoke at the Pete Gross House on a mission. The weather was cooperative, warm and sunny, and I slid on my Birkenstocks and took off on foot bound for Broad Street near the Olympic Sculpture Park. My route took me through the industrial section of South Lake Union that was early in its transformation to something more polished, and more to the liking of Paul Allen, the Microsoft founder who owned block upon block thanks in part to the laptop on which I checked email and updated the Carepage.

I passed Experience Music Project, Space Needle and monorail. A lot of Starbucks. Keys Arena was new since I'd covered Lakers-Sonics playoff games. I discovered arches that J and I had spotted from the Pete Gross House deck, and looked forward to telling her they were at the Pacific Science Center.

The large costume shop displayed nothing as scary as SCCA Transplant, and the options for temporary hair colors were sorely lacking. There was no blue. The proprietor said they'd sold out when the refs cheated the silver-and-blue Seahawks in the Super Bowl and turned all Seattle faces blue. She did have purple, the color of the UW Huskies, and I bought a can, just in case, then walked to another store downtown in search of blue. No luck.

I stopped in a Borders and bought Springsteen's *Seeger Sessions* and Karen Armstrong's *Great Transformation*. Armstrong's grasp of the ancient human desire to know God is compelling. I also bought one of those sticky rollers that remove hair from garments. My methods needed help.

The cut and coloring went well. J got to do some of both and had a ball. Then J let Amanda trim her mats, for starters, and then the rest.

I had a purple mohawk with a bald spot. I wasn't wild about the look, but I liked the effect. I got looks. Some with laughter. Some with knowing smiles. I like knowing smiles. I probably don't know what I think I know, but still.

Jody posted that J "looks absolutely stunning (Sinead, eat your heart out). With no hair on her head, her long lashes and dark eyebrows and big, sparkly, blue eyes pop out even more. A beautiful angel. But J doesn't think so right now. She's still getting used to it. Doesn't like to talk about it much. She's getting a lot of use out of all the hats we have collected."

J told Dr. Andrews about Boston and her nanny Penny, with whom she enjoyed myriad adventures the first three years of her life, while I worked long newspaper hours and Jody closed in on her Ph.D. "I got to know every inch of that place," J said. She also said she was eager for her new Lego set to arrive.

Legos are great, doctor said to patient, but neutrophils would get her out of the hospital. What Dr. Andrews didn't understand was, J had a sunny room big enough to park a Hummer in, a garden view, a bed with a magic wand and the daily attention of Left Coast Brooke and other nurses she loved. She was not clear why she should look forward to leaving.

Rounds became uneventful and routine. Other than the counts taking their time, everything determined by the daily blood draw was positive. Organs were functioning normally. Chemo sickness was over. She was eating, drinking and gaining weight. She had energy. Even J's angst over air bubbles in her Hickman line had diminished. Jody and I said something about not trusting the progress, about waiting for the other shoe to fall, and Dow just smiled and said this was why transplant docs love aplastic anemia.

Those might have been his exact words: *Transplant docs love aplastic anemia.* It's because transplant can go so predictably and smoothly. For all the concerns before and after, none involved wondering whether the cancer had been eliminated or would return. There was no cancer to begin with. If such a disease can be a blessing, the blessing is in the phrase, *It's not cancer.*

Awareness of this distinction and the pioneering approach to transplant for aplastic anemia had convinced Jody and I to move our faith cross country, and as Dow recounted the positive signs of normal organ function and minimal chemo reaction, I began to feel that maybe we'd made a profoundly smart decision for J. The stem cells still hadn't kicked in, and there were other things to watch for, and maybe always would be, but we'd somehow made it to this positive and promising place. I felt such exhilaration, joy, humility and gratitude for the people in Boston and Seattle who'd gotten us this far.

J raised her bed to nervous height and sat there munching on strawberries, Fritos and water. She was eating and drinking well enough to be taken off IV fluids. That Fritos were OK with the doctors took me back to the early days of her immune abandonment, when popcorn was banned for its kernels along with any kind of chip that might cut her gums. Those were days spent in fear of J's own mouth. And here she sat, riding high, munching on crunchy fun food without a care or a neutrophil.

I wasn't thinking about Graft Vs. Host Disease. Not yet. I was in too good a mood.

I posted about the arrival of neutrophils. J found it lacking, and offered her own: *"So my version of this story, and this is more accurate because I was the one who got up so early, NOT my dad. So, I was lying awake in bed, the sun had not risen yet, and Mom was not yet awake. Brooke comes in and she comes over to my bed, realizes that I'm awake, and says your ANC is 192. And I think, well, she wouldn't be just telling about the regular red blood cell count or platelet count, which I already have some of, so it must be neutrophils that have arrived. So, while I'm thinking that, Brooke opens up her arms and we give each other a huge bear hug. And I say, You did it Brooke! You brought them with you to my room! So Brooke says, be sure to let your mom sleep and not wake her up immediately and tell her. But of course, that's impossible, because Mom always sleeps in. So as soon as Brooke goes out of the room, I wait a few minutes and then say, Mom, and she says (in a groggy voice), What is it? and I say: Neutrophils are 192, and she says, You're kidding! And I say, No. And she says, Go back to sleep. That's my story."*

At the risk of destroying any remaining credibility regarding what constitutes a thinking man, a scene from *Finding Nemo* informed and moderated my overprotective instincts. In the film, Marlin is the widowed father on an epic search for his lost son, Nemo, and Dory is Marlin's sidekick who suffers from severe short-term memory loss. All are animated. All are fish.

Marlin (voice of Albert Brooks): I promised I'd never let anything happen to him.

Dory (Ellen Degeneres): Hmm. That's a funny thing to promise.

Marlin: What?

Dory: Well, you can't never let anything happen to him. Then nothing would ever happen to him. Not much fun for little Harpo.

The pods on Transplant connect something like a DNA chemical structure model. This makes for a challenging cart race course, so long as you watch for kids attached to IV poles, other kids on bikes and trikes, and nurses and staff carrying chemo bags or pushing carts or buckets of soapy water with mops. J, who grew up with a fast-walking nanny and a stroller on the mean streets of Boston, knew about sharing the road with pedestrians.

After a number of tours of Transplant on her pedal cart, J had a bright idea. She wanted to borrow one of the nurse's wheeled chairs, tie it to the chassis, and have me tow her, like a skier behind a powerboat. It seemed a bad idea to me, overly risky amid the ongoing platelet dearth. But there was no opposition to it among staff, or from Jody, and if they were OK with it, what was the guy with the vaguely purple stripe on his head who once approved helmetless sledding supposed to say?

We strapped on helmets and took off on a ride, and it was a hoot. We tested turns, to see what speed J could tolerate on her chair, how much she'd swing out left or right around a corner. Nurses thought it was hilarious. J thought it was hilarious. Doctors thought it was great exercise.

The cart was a striking machine—blue frame, big black tires with red rims, adjustable red seat. Other kids wanted a turn, but approval was specific to J, and we couldn't share. Another patient and her sister followed us around on foot. J was ecstatic. We toured every hallway repeatedly, lap after lap, back and forth past the play area, past the lead room for internal radiation therapy, past doors and curtained windows that never seemed to open, past sad eyes and smiles and name after name on door after door.

One shared room caught my eye. J and I shared a laugh, and I told a nurse that the paired names weren't sending the optimal message: Moore & Payne. She didn't get it right away, but as J and I pedaled away, we heard her howl, and we chuckled again.

Early during our stay on Seven West in Boston, with J's platelets in short supply, we saw a mother wheeling her child down the hall standing on the lower rung of an IV pole. J thought that looked like great fun, and talked me into trying it. As we rolled down the hall, a wheel hit a heparin cap or something and stopped like a shopping cart on a pebble with a jolt that felt like 6.5 on the Richter Scale. J began falling before I caught she and the pole.

The incident scared J. Me, too. The need for fun was secondary, but not unrelated, to the need for healing. Eight months later, in a different time zone and frame of mind, we hooted it up and zipped down the halls. Things had changed.

We wore helmets. Things hadn't changed that much.

We were back on the CBC roller coaster. We'd get one day's set of numbers and try to keep our emotions in check as we anticipated the next day's. "We can't all get too excited," Jody posted. "because the docs say it is normal for this number to fluctuate a lot. So tomorrow it may be 0. And the next day up again. But the docs are very encouraged and so are we. The marrow is settling in, I guess. But the thing that excited J the most today is that her online order of Legos arrived. Harry Potter's *Graveyard Duel* has upwards of 200 pieces, I think. She'll probably be through by tomorrow morning, assembling it. She is in heaven."

Encouragement was in potential revealed, not safety net created. Hundreds of neutrophils meant production. Five hundred or more could get us out of the hospital. We could really get excited, as Dr. Shannon had said, when one thousand became two thousand. With an ANC in the thousands, and time to mature, that prolifically snotty-nosed toddler on an Edinburgh bus could stop making like a Stephen King psycho in my memory and become, once again, merely disgusting.

On May 4, J's counts showed an increase across the board. This had not happened since the onset of aplastic anemia. They'd never all risen at once.

J was back in production.

The trend was sufficiently positive that Dr. Andrews began discussing discharge, and gave us a two-hour pass to take J on an outdoor adventure. It was her first time off Transplant since April 8. We got J SPF'd and drove to the UW Horticulture Center. J wasn't excited about the outing until we'd hiked to the marsh, where we counted 10 turtles sunning on the same log. We spotted redwing blackbirds, and then a great blue heron in performance. The nutria count was zero. The waters of Lake Washington sparkled.

Seattle Children's dedicated its new ambulatory care wing to Bill Gates' mom. We only got dial-up in our room. I found this ironic and funny; Jody and J, not so much.

PBS' *Now* did a negative report on the health insurance company whose policy we cancelled not long before J became ill. We might have had insurance headaches on top of J's illness. But Tufts insurance had made it easy and painless. We were lucky.

Dr. Andrews' rotation was ending. We'd relied on him for guidance, reassurance, perspective, and knowing what to do and when. He was a calming presence 24/7. He hung out with J, posed for a photo with her, introduced us to the new attending, Dr. Manley, who had been at Dana-Farber for a time before landing in Seattle. He had a tough act to follow. We hated to see our security blanket walk out the door.

But we'd follow Dr. Andrews out soon. We stopped waiting for neutrophils. Dr. Manley ordered GCSF, or granulocyte colony-stimulating factor. These proteins, produced in the human body, can be injected to boost production. GCSF had failed us in Boston, but we gave them a chance at redemption. J balked at another poke, but within a day of the onetime dose, her ANC cleared 2000. Dr. Shannon said we'd have a day like this. We started packing.

More than leaving, J looked forward to an arrival. Cousin Emily was coming from Boston. J wanted to create something befitting the occasion. So I squeezed a purple greeting on her bald head from the leftover tube of hair color. When Emily walked through the door, J lowered her head and removed a cap for the unveiling: *Welcome Em*.

J explained Emily to her Aunt Wrapping Paper. "Emily is kind of like my guardian angel," she said. On day 26 post-transplant, Emily arrived. On day 27, J was discharged. A guardian angel indeed.

On discharge day, we learned Molly O'Neill had been diagnosed with leukemia. Her parents were regulars on our Carepage, and close friends with Kristin. Soon they'd have their own Carepage, and be getting to know J's nurses and doctors in Boston. Molly was one of Emily's closest friends. I wondered what Emily, the child who opened my eyes to J's illness, was making of all this: her cousin bald and now with someone else's blood in her, her close friend suddenly with a blood cancer and harsh treatment and uncertainty ahead.

On discharge day, J's counts were jaw-dropping: 160 platelets, 2,200 ANC, 3,300 white cells, 'crit in the 30s. She'd been without a fever since November. Anxiety and uncertainty lay ahead, but nothing like before. Nothing like before.

On discharge day, I received a Carepage update. Amelia Quinn's mom wrote that she'd visited Jacob Noddy at Boston Children's shortly before he'd died in his parents' arms. Jacob had brought a cribbage board to Amelia at her funeral. I can see him at the casket like I was there, but I was thousands of miles away. Jacob was J's age.

There used to be entire days of unqualified good news. I miss them.

Like Seven West, SCCA Transplant became a family cocoon. The experience of leaving Seven West prepared us for the transition to outpatient care in Seattle, and our success getting J to transplant without a serious setback buoyed our confidence as we moved to the Pete Gross House. And yet, doctors weren't coming to us anymore. Nurses weren't knocking on our door and checking on us. We went from extraordinary 24/7 hospital care to seeing the doctor once a week.

We adapted. We hadn't a choice.

I posted: *"So J and I were playing Bingo on the living-room floor of our sun-drenched Seattle apartment when she suddenly decided to go head-over-heels. She came upright rubbing her head. The problem with being bald, she said, is when you do a somersault, there's no cushion."*

The good thing about platelets is, you can do the occasional somersault.

Jody asked our new outpatient fellow the elephant-in-the-room question: Was aplastic anemia officially a thing of the past? He said it was. What was the new diagnosis, Jody asked. He shrugged: "Normal." He said J was pretty much the ideal transplant patient.

We weren't sure we were hearing what we were hearing. Failed treatment teaches you to to dismiss or distrust good news. You get the answer you've prayed for, and you wonder, *What is he not telling us?*

A few minutes later, our new attending physician was almost apologetic that he didn't have more to tell us. When everything is going well, there isn't much to say. "See you in a week."

As Kristin and Emily returned home, Gerry and Lucy arrived.

"Here's the great news of today," J posted. "Are you ready? Here it is. Be prepared. I'm almost done with *Harry Potter and the Chamber of Secrets* (the book). Plus my Grandma Lucy bought me a Harry Potter reading light, so I can read in my bed at night. It's called the Lumos Book Light.

Lumos is a spell in Harry Potter that makes your wand light up at the end. The book light works terrifically and it casts a ghostly, spooky light across your page.

"Me and my Grandma Lucy and Grandpa Gerry went to see the new Seattle Library. And we used the gift shop as a total shopping spree. I got a miniature glass puzzle and a book mark for my dad and a new wallet for my mom. The wallet says, HMM, I WONDER WHAT I'LL BUY TODAY on it. I also got an umbrella that was completely unexpected, and we also bought the new movie *Harry Potter and the Goblet of Fire*. We watched it, and I got petrified. My head was spinning when it was over. I prefer *Harry Potter and the Chamber of Secrets* myself. My blood counts today are very good.

"The bookmark that I got my dad is carved out of wood and has a carved fern on it. My Aunt Mary Jo (aka Aunt Wrapping Paper) is going to be a grandmother for the second time. Her oldest child (Bill, my godfather) and his wife Elena are going to be parents again. Their first, Will, just turned two on Sunday and is going to be a big brother. That's all for now."

Had we been under water, I'd have been treated for the bends.

Seattle made up rainy and gloomy to keep people from moving there and overcrowding the place and turning it into L.A. *Don't come! Don't even visit. You'll get bummed out. Look what happened to Cobain!*

My Seattle basks in sunlight. It had been an especially wet winter, and the payoff was lush foliage and spirit-lifting rays. You could walk through any neighborhood, snap off a twig of rosemary, roll it between your hands, and then cup them to your face and breathe in the scent. Didn't matter what street you walked down, the rosemary would be there. It's like wild fennel in Spring in the foothills of Santa Rosa.

Out of the hospital, we had no commitments other than J's appointments. Her counts were inching upward, she hadn't needed a transfusion of red cells or platelets since late April, and even her cyclosporine levels were playing along. She was eating, growing, and had energy. We needed to limit her sun exposure, and went through tubes of sunblock finding one she didn't hate. We never did find that one, but some were less hateful than others. She didn't like hats. Another good thing about bald heads, they lend themselves to the thick application of lotion. Jody found SPF shirts online.

We bought a season's membership to the Japanese Garden. We visited the less manicured, more natural Kubota Gardens south of Seattle for a comparison. We liked both. The zoo, aquarium and swimming anywhere remained banned. So did crowds, but we frequented the massive REI flagship store during off hours, and J fantasized about having a turn on the indoor climbing mountain.

Eager to take J up the Space Needle, Jody got me as far as the lobby. We went at opening time, on a weekday, in the hope the crowd would be minimal, and a mask and Purell would be sufficient protection. We surveyed the crowd. Jody and J deemed it minimal. I got out my veto. Sometimes scaredy-cat wears like SPF-45.

We became regulars at a neighborhood park a short walk from the Pete Gross House. The community gardens, alive with butterflies, flowers and diverse imaginations, were fun to poke around in. We played tag using the passageways of the jungle gym for our escapes. But during recess at a neighborhood elementary school, it became the Park of Demon Children.

Immune suppression engenders fear of the sweet and innocent. It turns the nicest child into Draco Malfoy. We timed visits around recess, but you can't prepare for unscheduled arrivals at a public park. It was disheartening to time a trip badly, begin to have a little fun, only to flee a sudden swarm. With liberal use of Purell, J could play after they'd left, but not while they were there. The arrival of the swarm always put a disappointed look on her face. She resented them. So did I.

But there were successful, uninterrupted trips to the park, by ourselves, and with visiting siblings, parents, cousins, Jody's colleagues affectionately known as Psycho Moms. Each was a blessing and foretold a future without limit. J became adept on the monkey bars. We promised the doctors she wouldn't swing upside down or otherwise put herself at risk of injury. The Hickman was safe and snug under her shirt as she swung from bar to bar. The hat wouldn't stay on, but we SPF'd some more and took our chances. The monkey bars were making J's arms strong. Not strong enough to fend off the Malfoys, but strong.

Jody and I were aware of our comparative good fortune. Siblings or children of patients become lost in the chaos and stress of a life-threatening illness. We'd seen families split, one parent with the patient, one with other kids, miles or time zones away. In Boston, one woman staying with her son on Seven West had another child two floors up with a marginally lesser problem and wondering why Mom wasn't with him. This is where the Hutch School was magic.

At the Hutch, neglected children became the center of the universe. For a few hours they didn't compete for attention or feel guilty for wanting more. The Hutch School was an oasis, with teachers tailoring sessions to their psychological, spiritual and educational needs. A benefit is the burden it lifts from the patient. What this contributes to healing is immeasurable.

J couldn't attend classes. Her new immune system was both immature and suppressed by cyclosporine, which left her vulnerable. So she was privately tutored in the afternoons by Eileen, who became aware of J's interest in Mount Everest and geography. They printed out text and images of Norgay and Hillary and Tibetan flags, and prepared a presentation on the subject complete with detailed poster. J scaled Everest, Norgay and Hillary at her side, without ever leaving the Hutch School. She also dreamed of the climbing wall at REI.

In-patient and out, science enveloped J. Dr. Bender invited her to his lab at the Fred Hutchinson Cancer Research Center, across the street from the SCCA building. We went on a weekend when the building was near-empty. Bender met us as the door, ushered us past the Nobel Prizes on display in the lobby, and on up to his lab, where there are no Nobel Prizes but space is available. J spotted a poster on blood's myriad components, and Bender fed her fascination with an explanation only he could have made.

Jody wondered about other ways to feed J's interest in science, and Bender directed her to Penny Pagels, whose day job was educating science teachers in the public schools of Seattle. She agreed to tutor J. She refused payment. She and J hit it off and began a twice-weekly scientific collaboration in a room of the Hutch School.

Under the roof of the Pete Gross House, and the broader shelter of the SCCA, we'd found a home, possibly a cure, and an appreciation for the fullness of life. I'd worried that J's illness would create a dark space in her young life. But there was no void. There was illness and treatment and pain and suffering, but there also was remarkable attention to the things besides blood that sustain a life.

Jody gets the credit. She imagined, devised and created. She was diligent and enterprising, and left nothing to chance in creating opportunities to transcend our daughter's isolation. She was just as imaginative, diligent and enterprising in finding ways to keep the demands of J's illness from creating a void in our marriage. She's a treasure.

I posted: *"Things continue to go wonderfully for us in Seattle. We have a remarkably healthy, happy child, with much to be grateful for and look forward to. But this message is written with a great deal of sadness. Today my Carepage update brought word that Roy Ireland's doctors have run out of ideas. Roy is on a ventilator with myriad problems, and his family has run out of hope. His parents have made a decision no one should have to make. And boy do I wish I could do something for them during their last day with Little Roy. I got to know Roy's mom a bit while we were at Seven West, but not well. Seemed like every time we'd start a conversation, Roy would demand his mom's attention. With all the craziness that had befallen him, he didn't like competition for the person who was holding his world together. I sure couldn't blame him. As the songwriter John Prine wrote: Just give me one thing I can hold onto. So say a prayer for Amelia and Jacob and Roy and the broken hearts they leave behind. Be grateful for nurses and doctors and donors who make miracles happen with sick kids like they've done with mine. This moment is everything. Go find somebody to hug."*

Days were built around doses. Thank God for those M&M's.

It helped that J could swig the pills down with pulp-free OJ, which she loved, but then OJ was banned as J's potassium spiked, putting her heart at risk. Other banned foods were bananas, carrots, milk, yogurt, tofu, black beans, avocado, tomato, potato. I figured a little OJ with the meds would be OK, but then the next test showed the potassium higher still, and we were sent home with a prescription for Kayexalate, which lowers potassium suddenly, spectacularly and frighteningly, with a flavor deserving of a Bertie Bott's jelly bean alongside booger and earthworm and vomit. J took it once. It took longer going down than returning, and she refused to take it again.

I called the SCCA clinic, pleaded for an alternative, and the attending physician had an idea. He prescribed the diuretic furosemide, a quarter pill once daily, along with lots of fluids, especially water, but not OJ. I told J she needed to slosh when she walked. Her pill count now was 26 1/4, the highest she would reach, but the furosemide worked like a charm.

The potassium episode underscored that if I did what the doctors told me to do, I could keep J out of the hospital. But the priority changed like the wind, and beginning in Boston with the torturous days of feast and fast, I felt like Charlie Brown, except Lucy moved not the ball but the goalpost.

In spring 2006, the *New York Times* published an excerpt from "The Omnivore's Dilemma," the Michael Pollan book. Pollan endeavored to have a direct hand in what went into his mouth. He wrote of hunting pigs in Northern California. No Trader Joe's prosciutto for Pollan. There were graphic and disturbing aspects to the story. Then J said she was hungry, I put the magazine down and cooked some store-bought bacon. J loved bacon, and it has no potassium.

I'm not one for daily blessings at the dinner table, but I said something about the meaning of the Pollan story, with regard to the Native American ethic of acknowledging food's source and feeling and expressing gratitude. J said it sounded like a lecture. I do have a way of taking on the Voice of God.

They say people can take a long time to eat normally after transplant.

J posted: *"Today I went on the monkey bars THE WHOLE WAY! My dad was very proud. He has never seen me do it the whole way before and I don't think I ever have done it the whole way by myself. Actually, I did it twice. I must say, my hands are killing me from all that grabbing work. It was my half-birthday last week. And Aunt Wrapping Paper is sending a package probably. She told me that on the phone. What I think is funny is, when she sent the half-birthday card, there were Saint Patrick's Day stickers! Of course, my aunt is cool in that way. I like the stickers very much. We've been to two Japanese Gardens in Seattle. The one we discovered just recently is called Kubota Garden. It has a moon bridge, lots of other bridges, some waterfalls, koi fish, ducks, ducklings, lots of tiny tiny narrow trails that lead to places beyond your wildness imaginations! I thought it looked something like Hogwarts grounds from Harry Potter. And now I'm disappointed I told my mom that, because now she thinks that I'm scared and wants me to not read Harry Potter during the night. In fact, I think I'll read some Harry Potter right now. Off to Hogwarts!"*

J was off to Hogwarts. I was reading *The Lost Painting* by Jonathan Harr, who traces the remarkable story of a long-lost Caravaggio that turned up in a Jesuit residence in Dublin. Key information in unraveling the mystery came from a Roman palazzo that had been in the same family for 400 years and held a trove of personal and historical information. A library organized the family's documents, legal, marital, financial, etc., going back centuries.

As I read Harr's telling, I thought of a conversation Aunt Wrapping Paper had with our uncle not long before he died. While they chatted, Uncle Mac tended to some paperwork. He told Aunt WP he was going through a stack of his parents' letters, going back to their courtship. Sitting in front of his fireplace, with this box hauled up from his basement, he would scan a letter, tear it in half, toss it into the flames, and move on to the next one, saving only the photos.

Aunt WP tried to talk him out of destroying the papers and letting her go through them, but he was thinking about his own mortality. He was the steward of a legacy of privacy. He'd be the last hands to touch the letters, the last eyes on them. Aunt WP was in Northern California, Uncle Mac in Calgary, Alberta, so there was no way to knock on his door and plead in person. Unknown McLean history went up in smoke. Answers to ashes.

Dad and Uncle Mac got along OK, better than their wives, but the brothers lived the better part of two thousand miles apart, and weren't phone people. But in Dad's retirement, Aunt WP began making a weekly call to Uncle Mac, and she'd say hi and chat briefly, then hand the phone to Dad. The brothers got to talking, and made a reconnection that was important to both of them. Each told stories the other had never heard and repeated stories neither tired of hearing.

In the late 1980s, I took Dad to visit his brother, and we sat one evening in Mac's Calgary dining room, drinking bourbon and rye, Dad more moderately than his brother and I, and we got to talking about Uncle Frank, their mom's brother, who had taught Dad to drive. One day Uncle Frank up and disappeared, leaving behind a wife and young daughter, and Dad never knew what came of him. I got so caught up in Frank's story that I made one up. I wrote a novel. It's sitting in a box in my office. The true story's better, but I knew only fragments of it.

The weird thing was, Dad surprised his brother by saying he didn't know what came of Uncle Frank. Uncle Mac walked to his hall closet, and from a shelf above the Mister Rogers-style cardigans and a brown leather jacket I would inherit, he fished out an old shirt box and found a British Columbia newspaper clipping with a feature story on Uncle Frank from the early 1980s. Frank lived a long life, and Dad was both thrilled by the information and embarrassed that he hadn't known. Turned out, all he'd needed to do was ask his brother.

Uncle Mac let Dad have the newspaper clipping, which is a good thing. Now I have it. But I don't think Uncle Mac liked me writing about his ancestors, even in a fictional way. The letters went into the fire.

Dad did some genealogical research in his retirement. A cousin in central California fed him missing pieces, and he traced his McLean roots to John McLean Sr., born in Scotland in the mid-1700s, and who emigrated to Canada around 1790 with his wife and family, and farmed Lot 55 by the Cardigan River in Prince Edward Island.

My father's blood line continued with John Jr., then Duncan, then Stephen, my great grandfather, sixth of 11 children. Stephen worked in Boston, then took ill and went to PEI to recover but died instead. His son Reginald Joseph, my father's father, married Margaret Mooney from Glasgow, Uncle Frank's sister, and the proud woman who died with a purple face.

Dad stayed with her in the hospital in Calgary instead of driving with me for a round of golf at Banff Springs. Cancer cost us Saint Andrews, too.

The genealogical line is insufficiently drawn, but Dad was certain it reached back to Duart Castle. There'll be a Google Maps for DNA before I'm an ancestor.

I'm not sure how to describe the chain from John McLean Sr. to my father to me to my daughter. They are J's ancestors, and she has their DNA in her bones, but they are not her blood line. Not anymore. Her blood line belongs to strangers, who have stories I've yet to hear, like the ones that disappeared into Uncle Mac's fireplace.

I used to care, Dylan sang, *but things have changed.*

May 30 was Jody's and my 14th anniversary. She posted: *"We have much to be thankful for. We even had a date (!) while J was at school today. J surprised us with a gift of a snow globe with photos of our family inside."*

In a resource room in the lobby of the SCCA building, patients and families can check to see who has expressed mercy today. Sometimes it's a museum, a theatrical or dance company, sometimes sports, the zoo or the aquarium. I got two tickets to a Mariners game and invited an old friend from high school who'd relocated to the Northwest. We'd been in touch since our arrival but hadn't found a time to connect. The Mariners game did the trick. They played the Angels.

In our youth, when I was oiling my Brooks Robinson glove and wondering why my parents thought Bo Belinsky was a bad role model, Kurt was developing film and running cross country. Our friendship was never about baseball.

Kurt is of Japanese descent. His parents and grandparents were in Manzanar during the Pearl Harbor era before either of us was born and when West Coast America was afraid of all things Japanese. Manzanar was the Guantanamo of its day. Aside from the Jewish man who showed me the numbers on his arm at a bris in West L.A., Kurt's family were the only people I ever knew imprisoned for who they were.

While he and I grew up, America moved on with things, and we lived a sheltered life in an L.A. suburb and fancied ourselves open-minded and tolerant. Kurt married a woman widowed with two kids. I knew her late husband from high school. He was one of three brothers who died young from leukemia. No wonder E. Donnall Thomas, with his beagles, became obsessed with figuring this out. *Want to build me a wall so high nothing can burn it down,* Springsteen sang.

Kurt was an accomplished photographer before digital technology rendered his old-school talents as valuable as my ability to type fast on an Olivetti. Now he's an executive with a technology company involved with K-12 schools and student records. Times change. Kurt adapted well.

He and I sat in a private box, with tickets donated by a local business that didn't have clients to entertain for a night and wanted to do something nice for the cancer families. An SCCA van delivered us to the stadium and returned us home afterward. We watched a Japanese superstar play right field for the Mariners. He had three hits, was cheered loudly, and the Mariners beat the Angels. Our country had moved on to suspecting Mexican immigrants and Muslims.

Something about transplant increases a man's appreciation of tolerance.

J and I were playing with marbles from Aunt WP, listening to Springsteen's tribute to Pete Seeger, and suddenly J got this confused look. "Why is he singing provolone?" I laughed for the better part of a minute, then asked what she meant. She told me to wait till the chorus came around again. "Here," she said. The words are supposed to be: "Hold on, hold on. Keep your eyes on the prize, hold on." Bruce somehow made cheese of it.

I'm from the generation whose parents couldn't understand the lyrics, and now my daughter can't understand them.

Itching to be home, Jody was counting again. In early June we reached Day 62 post-transplant. We'd expected to return near Day 100, but a notable change takes place on Day 80 that is perhaps more definitional than anything. Day 80 is when the transplant docs stop looking for symptoms of *acute* GVHD and turn their attention to the *chronic* form of the disease. We had experienced no GVHD at all, which was remarkable. We had understood the likelihood that transplant would, at best, trade aplastic anemia for GVHD, but we had somehow managed to avoid GVHD in any recognizable form.

Jody began to query and lobby the transplant team about clearing us to leave early. J's remarkably good condition and the fact we would resume care at the Jimmy Fund Clinic were in our favor. And yet I was in no hurry to leave. When the Seattle doctors were ready, I'd be ready, and I had no interest in coaxing ourselves out of their care a moment before.

Besides, staying through the Fourth of July meant we'd have the best view in the city of fireworks over Lake Union and the Space Needle, right from our living room and balcony.

We got to know Lake Union well when we got to know Rick and Lewjean. Friends of Jody's aunt and uncle, they had relocated from Brookline to Seattle and had an old fishing trawler docked a short walk from our apartment. Rick and Lewjean invited us for a Father's Day cruise. J wondered why there was no Kid's Day, but this fast became one. She got to captain the vessel, under Lewjean's watchful eye. J wrote: "Steering the boat was fun but I kept on getting off target. But Lewjean helped me and it was tons and tons of fun." We motored around the famous houseboats of Lake Union, west toward the Chittenden Locks, back past Gasworks Park and Dale Chihuly's glass studio, through Portage Bay and the Montlake Cut by UW and out to Lake Washington.

After passing under the floating bridge, Rick steered us toward the massive estate of Bill Gates. As we came closer, Jody saw someone following us with binoculars. Rick said Gates owned the houses on either side, too, and had a security team looking out for the likes of us. He had much to protect. We didn't get too close to shore, just close enough to admire the place and keep security alert.

Another time, I wouldn't have cared much about viewing a celebrity residence. In forty years of living in L.A., I never once bought a star map of Beverly Hills, though I'm forever jealous of an actress friend who catered on the side and once made margaritas with Springsteen in his kitchen while preparing for a party.

But in 35 days at Seattle Children's, we got a good taste of Gates' philanthropic work. I wanted to knock on his door and thank the guy. I hope he enjoys that Lake Washington sunset view. I don't begrudge him that. Acts of kindness are welcome in any size, but on a scale and with an impact such as we witnessed, they're breathtaking.

I received word that John Andrew Ross died. John was minister of music at our church. He had looked to be at death's door any number of times, but then somehow he'd be back directing the choir that Sunday. His musical gifts were the reason we found a spiritual home. The first time

Jody and I attended our church happened to be its annual gospel music service; that music, more than anything, brought us back.

John grew up with Langston Hughes as a houseguest, and was instrumental in making *Black Nativity*, with text by Hughes, a long-running annual celebration in Boston, and a tradition for J and her nanny. I was saddened by the news, but oddly relieved. The death was of an adult friend, who'd lived a life, not of another kid from Seven West.

The closer we came to returning home, and the more we came to believe and trust that J was cured, the more I stifled my excitement. I feared letting my guard down. We could still blow this. And when I'd tell people positive news, it was like I'd hit some *Back to Normal* switch, and they'd fast-forward to jubilant assumption. There was such an eagerness to be past where we were. I became reluctant to share positive news and learned to put anything positive into context.

J's system was essentially that of an infant, and needed time to mature, as did my confidence. Isolation would continue through the end of the year, and she wouldn't be freed by her doctors to return to school, church or other crowds until after the anniversary of her transplant. And though the clock had nearly run out on acute GVHD, the chronic form had no such constraints.

J and I waited in a crowded room for a blood draw. J didn't wear a hat. I smiled at her, and she shot me a look and said, "What?!" She had no self-consciousness about her bald head, and I had lost track of how many days we were post-transplant. I'd stopped counting. The positive days had blurred.

J's counts and production had been stable and in a good range since we left the hospital. It had been two months since she had needed a transfusion of any kind.

Sitting in our Seattle apartment considering fate, coincidence and serendipity, J blurted out a poem. I asked her to repeat it, so I could write it down and post it: "Just think. If I didn't get aplastic anemia, I never would have gotten a bone marrow transplant. And if I didn't get a bone marrow transplant, we wouldn't have come to Seattle. And if we didn't come to Seattle, I would never have gone to the Hutch School. And if

I never went to the Hutch School, I would never have met Penny. And if we didn't meet Penny, I would never have gotten all of these things to look at under the loupes. Things like pepper seeds, twig with fungi, the mystery bone-like thing, the spiky podlike thing... a penny. One of those seed pods that flutter from trees. A piece of bright orange netting. A piece of a sponge. Light bulb. And the most beautiful, a perfect, whole sand dollar. Just think."

Jody went to North Carolina for her sister's wedding. Andrea had sent the dress she'd hoped J would wear in her wedding, and Jody took J's picture in it and brought it with her.

Jody wanted to invite someone to come stay with us while she was gone, or at least to arrange some coverage by an SCCA volunteer, but I declined. A weekend of just the two of us was what the doctor ordered. We called Zeek's to deliver pizza. We went for a walk along the docks of Lake Union. We went to the gym when it wasn't crowded, and J read *Harry Potter* while I listened to Bowie and zipped along on the elliptical as payback for Zeek's. We watched *The Dog Whisperer.* We rented the newly released DVD of *The Chronicles of Narnia,* which neither of us had read, and were surprised when Aslan the lion was resurrected. I should've seen that one coming.

J posted: *"I have some good news. Well, it's kind of good, and it's kind of bad. My bone marrow aspiration was scheduled for July 6, and that is kind off good and kind of bad. It's good because I wouldn't have a sore hip for the Fourth of July. But it was kind of bad because I sort of like having bone marrow aspirations because of the medicine they use to put you to sleep. It is called propofol. It makes you feel kind of weird and you get knocked out in about two seconds. And now the bone marrow aspiration has been moved to July 3rd. That's kind of bad because I probably will have a sore hip for the Fourth of July, and it's kind of good because I'll get that nice medicine sooner. My mom is gone for the weekend because she is attending her sister's wedding, which I cannot go to because the celebration is held in North Carolina! But me and dad are getting on verrrrrry well."*

They said we could leave, *barring something unexpected.* That phrase ranks with *a three-hour tour* from the *Gilligan's Island* theme. Our final clinic visit was scheduled for Monday, July 17. We received clearance after J underwent another bone marrow aspiration and biopsy. *Ow.* The news was all good, and there was more: She could stop taking three of her meds right away, including the bear bile. Her organs had made it through this process remarkably well, there had been so sign of acute GVHD, and the doctors were decreasingly concerned about its emergence.

Melissa few out from Rochester, N.Y., to spend the Fourth of July with us. Melissa's friendship with Jody goes back to high school. A professional cellist, she played at our wedding.

By Independence Day, J hadn't had a transfusion in three months. Jody and J made a patriot tart, with whipped cream, strawberries and blueberries providing flag colors. We watched the musical *1776*. Then we settled in for the fireworks.

Were it not for the disease required of residents, the Pete Gross House would be the envy of all Seattle on the Fourth of July. Our apartment was particularly well situated for the show, with views of both the Space Needle and Lake Union pyrotechnics. It was like sitting at center court for a tennis match, only with fireworks. The night was chilly enough that mostly we watched from inside the apartment. But for a while, J sat on my lap on the deck, and we took in the explosions to our west and north, every last one a stem cell multiplying, and it required no imagination, with each percussive blast, to squint and see the castle receding further into the horizon in the distance.

I woke up early on July 5 to the sound of helicopters. I made myself a cup of coffee and snuck up to the Healing Garden to see what was happening. Heavy smoke rose from an area on the eastern shore of Lake Union. An old pier belonging to the National Oceanographic and Atmospheric Administration had gone up within hours of the fireworks, though the cause was said to be a short in an electrical line.

As I arrived on the roof deck, the firefighting activity was for the most part over, though fireboats were still shooting Lake Union water on the embers. The stench was strong and acrid, from the burning creosote-soaked pilings, and I worried about J's vulnerability to toxic fumes. But the wind remained steady from the west, and made the fumes someone else's problem.

Good Morning America went for the heartstrings. The Hutch School does extraordinary things for families in difficult situations, and it felt good to see those efforts celebrated. The story was movingly told and prominently featured Iditarod racer Susan Butcher and her family. We were interviewed. J nonchalanted her baldness, albeit in the third person: "OK. She's bald. Big deal." She said she didn't need to hide her bald head for the camera. I was proud of that. *GMA* reported J was being treated for cancer. We'd been clear that it wasn't cancer, but what are you going to do. The story was about an institution with *Cancer Care* right in its title. In such a place, cancer is assumed. Better they say it's cancer when it's not than for it to be cancer no matter what they say.

I got caught up in the World Cup. With France playing Italy in the final, I wished I was home watching with my Italian brothers-in-law. Jody and J weren't interested, so I went to the gym. On a Sunday morning, the gym was quiet. I was striding away with the Olympic Mountains in the distance and Dylan on the headphones when bald Zidane head-butted the Italian. The head-butt was replayed repeatedly. Bald head lowered and slammed violently into Materazzi's chest. *I would not feel so all alone.* I looked around, but no one else was there. I couldn't understand the act. *Everybody must get stoned.* What a way to end your career. What a use for a bald head. What a brazen assumption of platelets.

Over the next few days, I made repeated trips to the SCCA mailroom, which lets patients ship packages at a discount. We sent 20 boxes home that way. All but one of them made it. We never did find out what happened to the other box, or even remember what was in it. The shipper asked for a list of contents, but we couldn't come up with one. We didn't seem to be lacking anything. We were coming home with everything we wanted.

Jody posted: *"The doctors and nurses keep shaking their heads in wonder at how well J is doing. It is very unusual that she has not had any complications, hospital readmissions, or Graft vs. Host Disease. She still has a 20 percent chance of getting Graft vs. Host Disease. But we are very hopeful that even if she does get it, it will be mild and treatable. This is all so miraculous."*

An SCCA volunteer drove us to Sea-Tac in her truck. She worked for Starbucks. She wouldn't accept money. She accepted gratitude.

We took a Tuesday night red-eye flight to Logan. I thought flying late might mean fewer sources of infection, but I'm not sure it made any difference, and the doctors weren't worried about it, anyway, so neither were we. We fastened our seatbelts. We flew commercial.

I posted: *"When I was a kid, my mom performed a ritual whenever she walked or drove past a Catholic church. She would bow her head and make the sign of the cross. The church was where God lived, she'd explain as she tugged on my arm and demanded that I bow my head and bless myself, too. For years, I thought I'd outgrown the practice. But lately, I've walked regularly (religiously, you might say) to the Seattle Cancer Care Alliance, a seven-story building that rises like a cathedral above the campus of the Fred Hutchinson Cancer Research Center, home to Nobel laureates and less recognized nobility, some of whom have been known to take hours out of their day to show a curious 8-year-old how science is done, and why. The SCCA building is rounded so as to envelope one upon arrival, and on a sunny day its windows reflect an expansive view of the shimmering waters of Lake Union. The place is a real sanctuary for those with cancer and related diseases, such as the severe aplastic anemia J suffered from when we arrived here. Suffered from. The past tense was never so loaded with future. Now, walking to the SCCA with J, or simply driving past, I don't bow my head or cross myself, but I do look up in wonder and gratitude for the men and women inside. I don't know where God lives, but I know where he works."*

CHAPTER NINE

Life in Positive Time

In late winter 2008, a photograph on the front page of the *New York Times* captured a scene from a village in China. A woman in a white apron worked in a drab room at a table covered in stacked buckets and pig intestines. Waste product spilled out of pots and over the side of the table. She was not making sausage, but beginning a process that would keep the life lines of humans from clotting. She wore a plastic sleeve over her arms, but I couldn't tell if she wore gloves, and I didn't see Purell.

She didn't work for me. Not anymore. The Chinese woman's distasteful task contributed to saving my daughter's life, but she was on to other children and adults, though I wonder if she even knew what she was contributing to. Some things it is better to know after the fact, or not at all.

Two years earlier, we were not past our need for heparin, and I am thankful that I did not carry with me then, as I injected the fluid into my daughter, the image of the woman toiling at the pig intestine table. The story accompanying the photograph detailed heparin contamination. The system had broken down, and the FDA seemed another watchdog turned lapdog. People died. In the hundreds of times someone's thumb pushed heparin into my daughter—sometimes it was J's own thumb, sometimes Jody's or mine— I never asked a doctor or nurse if the heparin was safe. I had no reason to question. I trusted.

The Chinese woman, slopping about under a fluorescent light, was in an initial stage of making heparin, which is extracted from the pig's mucous membranes. She would complete her work and hand her product off to a manufacturing and supply chain that would produce heparin's active ingredient and place it into individually packaged syringes and make it vital to saving human lives and worth a lot of money.

In Spring 2006, Jody was our specialist in the care of the double-lumen Hickman. Once you got the hang of keeping the Hickman clean, it was rather simple, really, except that if you screwed up or got lazy, the consequences could be awful, with J paying them, possibly with emergency surgery. She'd paid enough.

There was a routine to follow, and sanitary practice was crucial. First a cleansing daily shower. Then the various components of line cleaning would be arranged on a tray: disposable saline; alcohol wipes for flesh and lumens, packages torn at the corners for easy access; replacement IV connectors in case anything was dropped or otherwise put into question; sterile gauze and tape. We went through boxes of individually packaged wipes and sterile gloves.

J never took her eyes from a procedure, and became the resident Hickman expert. Jody evolved from practitioner to supervisor, at first because J wanted the responsibility, soon because she excelled. When I assisted, I backed J up with a checklist, but she did almost all the work carefully, attentively and flawlessly, one lumen at a time.

The last step, always, before gauze, tape and clean PJ's, was to flush the line with heparin. We went through boxes of individually wrapped and sealed syringes filled with the precise amount. I made sure we didn't run out, but didn't otherwise give a thought to the ready availability of the substance that was keeping the line free of clots and J free from the hazards posed by a clotted line.

The Chinese woman and her task wouldn't have interested me if it hadn't been for J's illness and the introduction to a new member of Maclean.org that arrived by email just after the transplant. I'd introduced myself to the extended clan not long before traveling to Scotland in August 2005, and every week or so I received bios of new members. In a brief bio, a woman said she was the granddaughter of Jay McLean, and that he had discovered heparin.

I'd never heard of Jay McLean and was unaware of any family connection. And yet the name was a powerful coincidence, and I wanted to know more.

I went online to learn more about him, and found a biographical essay by Jay McLean himself in Circulation, Journal of the American Heart Association, dated January 1959.

Jay McLean discovered heparin while looking for its opposite. That is, he wasn't looking for an anticoagulant, but studying thromboplastic substances that accelerate clotting. He was a second-year med student, and yet he was on a mission to prove his personal worth and solve a problem without assistance. "The discovery of heparin came as a result of my determination to accomplish something by my own ability," Jay wrote. "Just when this motivation arose in me, and what factors nurtured this determination ... are difficult to date."

Medicine was in Jay's blood. His father, John T. McLean, received his M.D. from University of California Medical School at Berkeley in 1867, and his uncle, Robert Armistead McLean, was "California's First Master Surgeon."

John T. McLean died when Jay was four. "A child knows when there is no breadwinner to rely upon," Jay wrote. Five years later his mother remarried. When Jay was 15, in 1906, the family home and his stepfather's business were destroyed in the San Francisco earthquake and fire.

Jay followed his late father and uncle to Berkeley, but wanted to research and teach surgery and saw his future at Johns Hopkins in Baltimore. The stepfather paid Jay's room and board at Berkeley but wouldn't or couldn't support the Johns Hopkins dream, which was further complicated by a Berkeley dean's letter to Johns Hopkins indicating Jay "was not the kind of man Hopkins sought."

Such was Jay's drive to become a doctor that he worked as a mucker at the Yellow Aster gold mine in the Mohave Desert, the gold bricks buying him a third year of college prep for Johns Hopkins. At Berkeley, he worked in the recorder's office, bookstores, scrubbing decks of lumber ferries, as a mail clerk on the railway from Oakland to Denver, and doing blood counts and urinalyses in the college infirmary. He was graduated from Berkeley in 1914, and finished with a bachelor of science and empty pockets, but even more committed to attending Johns Hopkins after studying a physiology text by William Henry Howell.

Howell was 30 years Jay's senior. He knew blood and how it coagulated like few in his day. Johns Hopkins rejected Jay's application, but he went anyway. His cousin, the anatomy professor Herbert McLean Evans, had just made the move in reverse, leaving Johns Hopkins for Berkeley, and advised Jay: "Ask no questions but look up for yourself what you want to know."

When Jay arrived at Johns Hopkins, the registrar "was surprised to see me and asked if I had not received the letter denying my admission. I told him I had, but figured on working a year; and I started to look for a job. The next day word was sent to me to see the Dean. I was informed there was an unexpected vacancy and I had been admitted."

Howell set him to work on thromboplastic valuation in a lab across from his own. Using brain tissue from a dog, Jay worked nights and weekends and soon was making progress on his research but not breaking into the department's inner circle. Howell and colleagues regularly went to lunch together. Jay wasn't invited. "I was not a colleague," he wrote. "This may also have been in part because my drying tissues produced an all-pervading insufferable odor which penetrated throughout the laboratory on the floor above!"

German chemistry literature led Jay to study cells of organs other than the brain, and he began comparative work on properties of the heart and liver. "The same process of extraction was used for brain, heart, and liver, yet in the brain, the end product was almost all cephalin, but in the heart and especially in the liver, it was something else which was mixed with cephalin."

Jay moved on to other research but put aside some cephalin and heparphosphatide for further testing. In time, what he saw in his serum-plasma mixture surprised him. He had been looking for what makes blood clot and stumbled onto the opposite effect.

About nine decades later, Jay's happy accident was keeping my daughter's catheter running smoothly and without incident. Indeed, the beauty of the discovery, and how others developed and advanced it through the 20th century, was evident in the remarkably uneventful nature of J's post-transplant days.

Heparin was part of why the physician's assistant could say, "Today is going to be boring."

Jay left Johns Hopkins to serve in the Army in France, but Howell continued the research with an associate and in 1918 published the paper that gave heparphosphatide the name heparin. Around 1930, a Swedish biochemist identified its scientific structure and readied the anticoagulant for testing. It was another five years before heparin came to be used in human patients at Toronto General Hospital, and a few years more before advances in tubing and dialysis transformed heparin into a life-saving fluid in the second half of the 20th century. In spring 2006, as J slowly, carefully and near-daily injected heparin into her catheter, the substance was among the oldest drugs still in wide clinical use.

I discovered another thing about Jay McLean. He declined Howell's invitation to co-author the historic 1918 paper in which heparin was described and named. "I had participated to such a small extent in this later work," he wrote, "and I did not feel entitled to the privilege offered."

I learned this from an anti-vivisectionist web page. McLean had proved heparin's anti-clotting potential on a live dog. Before my daughter's cure, before the nights on Heme-Onc and Transplant and fears of a clotted line, that might have offended me. *Things have changed.*

It was notable to Jay that he'd not been invited to lunch and treated as a colleague at Johns Hopkins. But when the invitation came to become a colleague, as co-author, he declined. His role was forgotten. Historical credit wasn't granted to him in medical circles until the 1940s, and with the posthumous publication of *The Discovery of Heparin* in Circulation in 1959.

Jay's remembrance of his discovery, written shortly before his death in 1957, is sprinkled with doubt and determination. That he would decline co-author credit for something that mattered so much to him is both strange and strangely familiar. Maybe it's a McLean thing.

My father was a humble man of great integrity, and his humility had a way of supplanting his ego. It's part of what made him so likable, and why I miss him so much, but I'm sure it limited him professionally. I'd love to see a list of things Dad denied himself so that I could have what I needed; I know it to be long. Dad's dream of becoming a medical doctor was sidetracked by the Depression, and he never completed his degree. Of the things he accomplished, I can't think of one driven by personal ambition.

An aptitude test from high school said I should become a pediatrician. I don't know what that test was thinking.

A grainy photo of Jay I found on the web looks more like Mom's father, an Irish O'Byrne, than my McLeans. I also don't know how closely we're related, or the precise number of times Jay's discovery was injected into my daughter's blood stream. Hundreds, certainly.

Jay McLean made life easier for countless kids, and adults, getting poked and cut and drawn and infused and anesthetized and organ-swapped and suppressed physically, spiritually and immunologically. He was an introspective man with a passion for his work but seemingly doubtful of his own potential. This is familiar, as if in the blood.

J and Victoria, friends since preschool, are budding scientists. They'd study life in the neighbor's pond for hours. Their discoveries often resulted in little more than *That's gross!*, but sometimes there was a more notable advance in understanding. They took good notes, and shared observations.

Sometimes my daughter downplays her talent as a pianist, but it doesn't stop her from advancing further into the Bach, Clemente or Scarlatti repertoires. She doesn't brag about it, but I don't think she doubts her talent or worth. I compliment her playing every chance I get, and I get lots of chances, with the prospect of many more. Thanks, in part, to heparin.

Jay McLean wrote his own story of heparin's discovery, about forty years after the fact, but never finished it. Cancer took him quickly, and he died in Savannah, Georgia, on November 14, 1957, at age 67.

The woman at the pig intestine table wouldn't even have noticed that lab smell, the one that cost Jay an invitation to lunch. I'd like to take both of them to lunch. Somewhere vegetarian, maybe. I'll bring the Purell.

Chapter Ten

Cry Silencing & Dog Whispering

Until J spiked her first fever in months, we'd not spent a night on Transplant at Boston Children's. Jody and I visited once, touring the sixth floor unit while sorting out where the transplant should take place. The rooms are small but private, the space warmly lit. Nurses and staff were as engaging as possible, but stopping to schmooze a prospective family is tough when a kid is due for another bag of cyclophosphamide and counting on you to cope with the after effects.

Admission is restricted, and a visitor must step through one set of doors, wait for them to close and seal, then push a button to open the next set and enter the cocoon. The air system is designed to maintain sterility. This is the bubble in the new normal.

A prominent plaque dedicates the ward to a physician whose name causes some Jimmy Fund parents to tear up in gratitude. She's a saint to them. More than a saint, she's a transplant physician. There are young adults alive because of magic she worked when they were toddlers. I know one of them. For us, she was the expert whose recommended treatment we turned from in choosing Seattle. She wanted greater proof that the Seattle protocol took J's illness seriously enough. That level of proof wasn't available yet. We found our proof wrapped in hope. We moved. Now we were back.

Aunt WP came east for a visit. Jody was catching up with the Psycho Moms and Aunt WP was hanging out with J and I when J began to sag. Her temperature was over 101. The transplant attending at Boston Children's said to pack a bag and come immediately. I suggested we wait, take another temp and talk again later, but the doctor said no. This was the formal handoff of care for another hospital's transplant patient. There would be no messing around.

The emergency doc gave J Tylenol—*Where have you gone, Dr. Shimamura?*—and her temp was back to normal before we were admitted

191

to Transplant. The Transplant attending came to meet us. The name was familiar, but she'd not met either of us before and needed to familiarize herself with our case. We talked about Seattle and the reduced TBI and research protocol, about the fact there'd been no hospitalizations since the transplant more than four months earlier, about the remarkable lack of GVHD. J's counts were fine, her ANC a staggering 3750. The calendar said they were immature and not to be trusted.

I asked the doctor about her last name: Janeway. I said J's late Grandpa David had trained at Boston Children's years earlier, and a Dr. Janeway had been his mentor.

I didn't know David as a doctor. By the time we merged into that hybrid blood line that includes in-laws and step people, his creative energies were directed toward environmental and scientific philanthropy, and later to pursuing the mix of psychological, spiritual and medical intervention that might postpone melanoma's death sentence.

I did get one real look at the pediatrician. David intervened as J's advocate when she was days old, barely five pounds, and Jody and I struggled with breast-feeding contraptions and strategies. J was having none of it, and hadn't the weight to wait. That was David's point in saying 'she needs calories now" and he didn't care how she got them. We went with formula, and J began to thrive. Weeks later, when J received the Hib vaccine, David wasn't at the appointment, but he couldn't have been more present.

David believed he could change the world, and he did. Any child born since about 1990 in the first world, and increasingly in the developing world, almost certainly will not contract what was the most dangerous cause of bacterial meningitis. There's a vaccine for it now, thanks to David, who if he were still alive and you were to ask him, would soon mention Charles Janeway, a driving force in the research that led to the Hib. David was J's grandfather, but they were related by fate, not blood. Then again, I'd argue that any child vaccinated with the Hib is related to David by blood. Long before any child was approved to receive it, David injected himself.

The last time I'd heard the name Janeway was in David's barn in Martha's Vineyard in September 1998. Jody and I sat with David, interviewing him on our pre-digital camera to preserve some of his story in his own words. He hadn't much hair; aggressive cancer treatment had rendered him gaunt and weak. But even a diminished David was no less driven to change the world or celebrate those who might. He told us about Janeway's influence on a career in medicine and science that resulted in the Hib vaccine in the 1980s.

When J received the Hib, delivered via nasty big needle, she wailed. I shook in awe. The pediatrician said to tell David thanks, and I passed those words along that day in the barn. David appreciated hearing it, but he turned the conversation to how scientists at UC San Diego were advancing the vaccine. He was excited less talking about the vaccine that didn't exist before he and his colleagues went to work than potential of successor scientists eliminating excruciating ear pain—silencing the cries in the night of children he'd never know, and perhaps allowing a child to one day grieve her parent's death, as it ought to be, and not vice versa.

David spoke so appreciatively of Janeway. One day during rounds, gathered around a child in agony, Janeway said, "Why don't one of you try and find a vaccine for this?" The man understood David, saw his potential, and helped direct him onto a path toward eliminating a killer of children.

Hib, short for Haemophilus influenza type B, causes meningitis, pneumonia, brain damage, and kills about a million annually in the developing world. It is transfered through the air in droplets. Children under 5 are especially vulnerable.

David told Jody and I about his collaborator Porter Anderson, whose protégés in Infectious Diseases would search in vain for the cause of J's fevers in September 2005. David died too soon, but to die knowing you've saved a human life, even one, what higher purpose might there be?

And yet I hadn't remembered the name Janeway until I saw it on the doctor's lab coat. J's fever came and went with blessed rapidity, but not so rapid as to preclude a 48-hour admission, these still being days of questionable immunity and taking no chances. Dr. Janeway checked J closely. And then I told her J's grandfather had been mentored by a Dr. Janeway, and asked might there be a connection? "He was my grandfather," she said.

She was taken aback by the connection and the story, but seemed to have heard versions before; the list is long of Harvard-educated doctors whose lives and careers her grandfather shaped. She smiled, and said she looked forward to telling her father. She was a third generation Janeway in medical practice.

Dr. Janeway, while attending to my newly afebrile daughter, was pregnant – with twins. I asked if she knew their specialty yet. "You can't say things like that," Jody tells me. "People don't understand your sense of humor." Dr. Janeway gave me an quizzical look, as she sorted out what I meant, and then she grinned. Then she called upstairs to see if J's room was ready.

Months later, Dr. Whangbo said Dr. Janeway and her newborns were doing well. I hope the twins' only experience of the Jimmy Fund is to visit their mom at work and maybe walk in the annual fund-raiser. Before long, they'd receive the Hib. Then Dr. Janeway could cross Haemophilus influenza type B off her list of things a parent worries about.

Dormant fears awakened in J. She knew a trip to the hospital could begin an unpredictable journey. She found herself in a new unit, without her trusted Seven West or Seattle nurses. Aunt Wrapping Paper was in town. Lousy timing. But what most disappointed her was that the cable system didn't carry the National Geographic channel, and it was *The Dog Whisperer* marathon week. She had looked forward to multiple nightly episodes, only to get cheated by a fever that went away faster than a poodle intervention.

The disappointment wasn't solely J's. Jody's and my obsession with *The Dog Whisperer* began in Seattle. As the patient's parent, you either sit around thinking about what it is that is causing the isolation, about your powerlessness and fear, about how it is you landed on the wrong side of *There but for the grace of God go I*, or you find ways to escape.

I loved the show, but even more I loved this fact: *The Dog Whisperer* features a man who snuck across the border from Mexico and became famous in America for teaching troubled dogs not to jump fences and go where they're not wanted.

Cesar Millan spoke to us loudly: *I rehabilitate dogs. I train people.* With no dog, just a cat, a guinea pig and the occasional toad back home, we gave ourselves over to Cesar anyway. Jody listed dates and times on a Post-it on the TV. One episode would end, and J would want to know when we could watch the next one. *More*, we begged, and in time Cesar would throw us a bone.

Back home, for J to find herself admitted to Boston Children's during a nightly marathon of *The Dog Whisperer*, only to learn the TV in her room couldn't get the show, was upsetting. We made the best of it.

The fever was brief, a welcome indication of an immune system more mature than the calendar gave it credit for, and J got to watch several episodes at home. We were watching Cesar and his pack work their magic that Saturday night when it was time for bed. I tucked J in, switched to CNN, and learned of Susan Butcher's death.

I wonder what Susan would have thought of Cesar's way with dogs. His methods can seem simplistic, and yet their effectiveness is undeniable and his love for the animals obvious. Cesar comes across as a strong, fearless man, but he tears up just about every time he scores some breakthrough with a dog and its family, and I can imagine his eyes moistening at seeing Susan with her pack. Cesar would not need to explain his concept of pack leader to a woman who four times won the 1,100-mile sled-dog race known as the Iditarod, nor would someone who once snuck across the border for work hesitate to cheer a woman upsetting the men's club.

I hadn't owned a dog since a purebred beagle named Maggie. A friend told my ex-wife the apocryphal story of beagles stolen for research, but Maggie was a victim instead of the failed experiment that was my first marriage. Cesar would have loved Maggie and given me a talking to. Among his clients, the behavioral problems are never idiopathic. The causes are invariably staring back at the camera from the incredulous eyes of the dog's owner.

Susan Butcher's husband was warm and engaging in those moments when our paths crossed—riding the SCCA elevator, sitting in a waiting room, or at the Hutch School, which their daughters attended. Soon after we arrived in Seattle, Susan shared a poem at a reading for Hutch children and their families. I could tell she was in treatment, or thought I could, but didn't otherwise know who she was. A couple of months later, a crew from ABC's *Good Morning America* came to the Hutch to do a story. Susan, the resident celebrity, agreed to participate.

Susan's family lived in Alaska but relocated to Seattle for however long it would take. It was of great concern to her how her dogs would be cared for while she was away. Friends came to the rescue. Susan had a powerful way of rallying people to a cause. She and her family brought countless new donors into the national marrow program, source of J's perfect match.

I never met Susan at her athletic and physical peak, but I might have met her at her most determined. She was on a Hutch School sofa appearing unable to stand up without assistance. The intensity of her gaze was missing. Still, she gamely attempted to lend her celebrity to the SCCA and the Hutch by granting an interview to *Good Morning America.* She was weak; the crew was patient. Her husband brought warm soup, and she was sustained. She sang with her daughters for the camera. She did the interview.

Perhaps three months later, as I watched CNN recount simple facts of Susan's life in reporting her death, the four Iditarod victories were noted prominently. There was no mention of the movement to end the Iditarod spearheaded by People for the Ethical Treatment of Animals.; it was not the time or place for that. Neither did the story go into how, for some, the Iditarod recalls the role of sled dogs in getting serum to a snow-bound Nome during a diphtheria outbreak in 1925.

Something else was missing from the CNN report, and so I went online to find an answer more specific than "cancer" to what doctors said had killed her. I found it in a wire service obituary: Graft Vs. Host Disease. Susan's first transplant did what it was supposed to do in eliminating the leukemia, but then the marrow revolted against its host. Another transplant was needed. The revolt continued. Susan died.

My daughter's life was saved by dogs. There was no pack trudging miles through the snow to deliver serum. There's Fed-Ex for that now. No, the dogs that saved my daughter's life have a more complicated tale, and it spans roughly my lifetime.

The medical community does not like to call attention to biomedical animal research because people don't understand it, and some actively oppose it as morally wrong, sometimes with letters to the editor or checks to PETA, sometimes with anonymous aggression. They make no distinction between research for vanity or humanity. They make big and violent statements and claim information derived from research involving animals serves no good purpose in treating humans.

I know this to be untrue.

I know of a doctor who had blood smeared on the door of his home for having the audacity to find ways by animal means to save human lives. He thought one was worth the other, and I thank him for it.

The home of a Los Angeles scientist investigating human nicotine addiction was flooded within weeks of a newspaper story mentioning her research involving primates. In claiming responsibility, the Animal Liberation Front said it had a tough time choosing between flooding and burning. Months later, they returned with a firebomb.

I can only assume the process that allowed medical science to save my daughter's life is considered morally wrong by people with unending compassion for animals. I don't understand this.

I never met E. Donnall Thomas, though I got in the habit of looking at his kindly countenance on the portrait prominent near the elevators at the SCCA clinic. Thomas' research with dogs resulted in a paper published in the New England Journal of Medicine in 1957, three years after my birth, that is considered seminal in the development of transplant.

J and Jody were not so caught up in the Thomas story, and I became something of a scold. "He's the reason we're here," I'd say, using what J calls my lecture voice, and in so many words asking them to bow their heads as Mom had instructed me when we'd walk or drive past a Catholic church. "God lives there," Mom would say. And so I'd repeat to my wife and child, "He's the reason we're here," when we'd pass Thomas' portrait, which hung like a saint in stained glass; Thomas the indubitable.

Now that I'm a bit more educated about blood and its history as a medical product, I'm grateful it wasn't in 1957 that someone I loved needed a transplant of bone marrow, because the outcome would not have been so positive. As recently as the 1980s, getting simple transfusions for a disease such as J's was essentially trading one problem for another. But in 2006, after years of transplant research involving mostly mice but also beagles, and vast improvements in the blood supply as a legacy of AIDS, J received significantly less pre-transplant irradiation, milder, targeted chemo, and a second chance at life.

Thomas won a Nobel Prize in 1990 for decades of research into bone marrow transplantation. He was courageous and visionary, but without his dogs, he would have been a scientist on a short leash, and who knows what would be my daughter's fate.

J, Katherine and Abigail set up an ice cream stand on our front steps. Our street's a dead end, but they raised 45 dollars for the Jimmy Fund. Afterward Jody told J to give her the cash and she'd write a check, but J thought that was a bad idea. She wanted the Jimmy Fund to have the actual money they'd raised, and to deliver it in person in honor of her friend Molly and her treatment for leukemia. Sometimes J fills me to bursting with pride. A lot of time, actually.

The ice cream sale led to another, which brought in more money, then to a bake sale, with J and her mom doing the baking, and that went well, too. Another time J had me fix smoothies. One neighbor passed on the smoothie but gave J 20 bucks. I could see J's mind at work. The stands never did so well when they were about raising money for herself.

Jody took J to deliver the money, not to the Jimmy Fund Clinic itself, but to the business office about a half-mile away. They caught the staff by surprise. Disconnected from the patients who daily pass through the clinic, the fund-raising staff wasn't used to transplanted children with donations in hand. They accepted the donation in Molly's name and proceeded to raid the supply room for goodies for J. They exchanged expressions of gratitude for good works and kind gestures, then J left to plan her next sale.

I posted: "*The interest in J's health journey amazes me sometimes. We're all amazed, as well, at the outpouring for Jody's participation in Sunday's Jimmy Fund Run. Jody had in mind to raise $1,000 for the Jimmy Fund. Well, one person alone took care of clearing that goal, and other family and friends are likely to get her past $5,000 by the time she starts cursing her blisters on Sunday. One of the generous contributors is my brother Ron in Southern California. He and his family have been a big support to us along this journey, and now Ron's about to begin his own battle with cancer. It isn't his first. Ron wrote: "I will begin my treatments next week, and will go at it with a J attitude." I ask all those who have contributed to our healing on this webpage to send a healing thought my brother's way. During our Jimmy Fund* *visit on Tuesday, J and I bumped into mother Leslie and daughter Sydney, our Seven West neighbors for weeks in Fall 2005. Leslie gave me a hug. She didn't give J one. She knows better. The smiles on mother and daughter's faces were something to behold. The Jimmy Fund works magic."*

We received a letter from the marrow donor.

"To my recipient and family;

"Thank you so much for your beautiful cards that you have sent me. I look forward to updates and I'm so glad that she's doing so well. Everyone I know is also very glad as they have been so interested in this whole process. Many people are praying for you and your family as you go through this. I'm so honored that I matched you and was able to donate so quickly. And I'm so glad that there have been so few complications. God is so good.

"Well I wanted to tell you some about me since you've told me so much about you and your family. I'm 25 years old and I'm in my fourth year of medical school. Med school has been a great experience for me. I plan on pursuing a career in pediatrics when I finish up this year. We find out on March 15, 2007, where we'll end up for residency and then I'll spend 3 years wherever that ends up being – hopefully in the same place that I am now. I got on the bone marrow registry through a blood drive at my school in January 2005. I was shocked when I got the call less than a year later.

"Before med school I went to a small college and majored in biology. I was also very involved in the band – I play clarinet. Before I went to college I also took piano lessons for 10 years, so I'm glad that my recipient loves music – it definitely was/is one of my favorite things. And I'm glad she likes science – she sounds a lot like me.

"Other than school I love to be with my friends, I love being outside (although it has been so hot here lately). I've gone on several medical mission trips – something else I love to do – and

I'm actually leaving again on August 11 to go to Kenya for two weeks. I'm excited about it although I still need to pack. I love being able to give back to those around me.

"Let's see, what else … I'm very involved in my church here – it's been a blessing to end up there for the past few years while I've been in school. I'm so glad to hear that you get to return home soon (you'll probably be there by the time you get this). How exciting that everything has gone as well as it has and you get to return home. I'm so happy for you. I look forward to hearing how things are going as you settle back in there. You are all in my thoughts and prayers often and I look forward to hearing from you again soon. I hope you have a wonderful rest of your summer.

"Best wishes to you and family,

Your donor"

His name was Pebbles, or maybe it was her name; it's hard to tell with robots. Pebbles was Smurf-blue, the same color as Dad's 74 Plymouth Valiant with the foam front seat that over time swallowed him up like quicksand and made him look like a tyke at the bank teller.

Pebbles is an acronym for something long and unwieldy and not terribly clarifying. He moved into our basement. A counterpart moved into J's classroom. Through phone line or broadband cable, Pebbles would be a port key for J to sample the life of a third-grader that she was missing.

My mom believed in bilocation, that there were saintly human beings of a rare and deep spirituality and divine connection who could be two places at once, and participate in a sort of mystical multitasking. Broadband would be cheating, but still.

Libby scanned her classroom, counting kiddos. *Abigail's here. Andy's not here. Ben's here.* She continued down the list. *Jeremiah's here. J's here. Maria's here.*

I cracked up. J shot me a look. But J was not *here* in Libby's Lincoln School third-grade classroom. J was *here* with me in our basement, and Libby was counting her as present five blocks away.

Our basement is something of a bunker. J liked me to stay while she was in class, and in the long and problematic process of making the robot more fruitful than frustrating, it was good that I stayed in close proximity. But it was difficult keeping my nose out, and now and then I'd nudge J to answer her teacher, to verbally acknowledge her classmate and not just shake her head, to stop daydreaming, to raise her robotic hand to let the teacher know to move the microphone so she could hear, to not simply get up and leave but tell the teacher she was taking a short break.

She'd shoot me the look. *Dad, this isn't your class!* The daydreaming concerned me, but the inconsistent connection to the classroom encouraged a tendency to drift. Besides, I'd been a classroom daydreamer with no robot to blame.

Lesson in session, kids working quietly at their desks, suddenly laughing and screaming *ick!* and *gross!* and evacuating the classroom. Everyone but Pebbles and us knew what was happening. Then a door opened, and J and I watched the janitor, oblivious to us, sprinkling what janitors sprinkle and doing what janitors do to clean up vomit. Soon, the teachers and all but one child returned. Libby apologized for forgetting us, but we were forgiving. Some classroom events are better experienced via robot.

Libby gathered the children around her in a half-circle, and began to read a story. The audio cut out. J sighed, raised Pebbles' hand, and let Libby know she couldn't hear. The teacher asked the boy sitting on the floor mike to move. Audio was restored. Later, J raised her hand again, waited to be called on, and said, *Miss Donovan, somebody's drumming on the microphone.* The teacher handled it with grace. Little Charlie Watts had been outed, embarrassed, and Libby didn't call attention to the offense. "We'll stop doing that," she said simply, and the beat ceased.

Next day, a kid who normally spoke inaudibly made himself heard with a cough that obliterated all remote attempts at learning. A wet, phlegmy croop one moment, a dry hack the next, then another thick and liquid cough. Maybe it was two kids. I found myself wanting some 9-year-old to sidle over and put a mask on the mic. Ridiculous, I suppose. Paranoid, perhaps. I was both.

This was only Libby's second year running her own classroom, and I'm not sure a more experienced, set-in-her-ways teacher would have given the robot the time and effort to make it work. She was inventing her own teaching style, making the school district curriculum fit her day-to-day, which was complicated enough without adding a blue plastic student with wheels and an umbilical cord. It's hard to say what her incentive was. I'm sure the goodness of her heart had a lot to do with it.

On Libby's first day in her own classroom, a child went out sick with a life-threatening illness; Libby went out of her way to bring that child back to school. And throughout the process of getting Pebbles up and running, she was patient and helpful. She educated herself about the robot, how to make it work for J, how to make it work for the entire class.

I'd feared the robot would be disruptive—the ultimate difficult student, sucking energy out of the room. But Pebbles was like a special needs child who with the right teacher, the right comprehension of a unique learning style, locates hidden talents.

Even before Libby, I had a soft spot for elementary school teachers. Aunt WP got her teaching credential a short while before her marriage ended. She had quite a career, and I marveled at her commitment while seeing her school district transition from high times to low. Affluent residents moved or paid to educate their kids in private schools. The public schools waved goodbye and placed their hopes on the lottery. Their number never came up.

Aunt WP and I watched the staggering achievement that was the California public education system shrivel in Proposition 13's aftermath like a California raisin. Property taxes shrank right along with the value of living there. About the only resources left for students in a public school system like hers are the Aunt Wrapping Papers.

The school system in Brookline is an oasis. Residents complain about taxes on a daily basis but pay them anyway and vent about it at Starbucks over a steaming $4 mocha. Beginning with her three years of preschool, J had learned to love learning, thanks to dedicated teachers. And yet, if it wasn't for Libby and the way she made J a member of the class via Pebbles, I could have been won over to home schooling. During her extended isolation, J's one-on-one educational experience with tutors was extraordinary, and opened my eyes to what was possible outside the classroom.

In Boston and Seattle, teachers filled J's missing second grade year with enlightenment and enthusiasm and even the basics.

Any daylight between J and her classmates, Susanne took care of. In a previous life, Susanne was Lucille Ball or a Marx Brother. Chico, probably. J spent 90 minutes with Susanne twice a week for most of her missing third-grade year. Their sessions were fun and full, and J would shoot me a look when I arrived to take her home.

They met in Susanne's classroom, across the hall and down from where a fully immune J should have spent the day. We'd allow time for the daily horde to evacuate the building, and for Susanne to disinfect a work table. J knew not to pick things up. We'd race through the school like the lobby at Children's, saying fast hellos to surprised faces as we zipped by. I'd drop J off and they'd get to work on addition, subtraction, spelling, science.

Meanwhile, with Julie, J was learning to love piano. She continued learning the benefits of yoga with Peggy. And one fall afternoon, she learned to ride her bike. For so long, lacking platelets, I wouldn't let her even try. Now, she had platelets, a helmet, growing confidence, and one day it just seemed to click. She made it a short distance, stopped and smiled. She went a few more feet, stopped and smiled again. In minutes she was riding the length of our dead-end street. She was proud. I called Ann Marie to tell her. Ann Marie had been J's tennis teacher from around age 5, and had encouraged her on the bike during breaks from tennis. J missed a lesson the day her symptoms arrived. When J would fall, Ann Marie would encourage her to climb back on. That's what a good teacher does.

Halloween was warm and dry, and J was OK'd to go trick-or-treating. Jody went with her. I sat on a bench on our front porch and handed out candy. Frightful creatures ascended our steps to ask for sweets and threaten untold acts. Many arrived with fake head wounds. I considered giving out platelets. Nobody'd get the joke, but still. J went as a surgeon in a hematologist's lab coat, a gift from Dr. Whangbo. Her mask was just part of a costume.

J was frightened by a neighbor's scary music. Given all she'd been through, she was still a kid, and this was a welcome reminder. She could still be frightened by things that go bump in the night. She was also still reassured that Jody and I could provide protection against dark forces. Go figure.

Sitting on the front porch, I was aware that this was the second All Hallows Eve since diagnosis. Halloween is a favored holiday for J. She can celebrate the fearful, then put the costume away, or even throw it away. That's a good thing to do with fears.

The surgeon was a joke cracker, witty, smart. Of course he was smart, he was a surgeon. But he was also a distinction in scrubs between intelligence and wisdom. With a hard, yanking motion, evidently to lighten the moment, he acted out how he would remove the Hickman. J wasn't amused, and neither was I. He may have been the sharpest tool in the drawer, but the metaphorical instrument for his wisdom was more ball-peen in nature and blunted by underuse. Having someone so edgy and dark interacting with a vulnerable kid is beyond me, like asking Severus Snape to put your child at ease.

The guy did amazing work with the knife, don't get me wrong. We'd had long days with surgery before, and this wasn't one. I give him credit for that. But in preparing a kid for surgery, he was as lost as Harry without his wand. J could have used Versed and propofol before meeting him. Me, too.

Maybe I resented the guy because he was removing my life line. The Hickman never entered my tissue or arteries, but became part of me. The Hickman generated its own fear during installation and for a while afterward, but for seven months we had cleaned it, cared for it, nurtured it, and I'd seen it transcend its plastic reality with countless, painless infusions and draws, and the very delivery of the donor's miraculous gift. It was external access 24/7, and I treasured it, held it up and consecrated it. Removing it was to watch the safety net disappear. They said we didn't need it anymore. *How did they know that?* I wanted conclusive proof that the Hickman wasn't going to be needed again. I wanted it written in Blood. *What happens if the counts plummet tomorrow? Then what?*

I hate seeing J in pain, and few things caused her pain and frustration more than having an IV shoved into her arm, hand or foot, and left there. The port solved that problem, and with Emla, timely applied, allowed for painless accessing. Still, I'd watched nurses approach J's chest with needles, count and shove, and I flinched every time. I thanked God for the port, but every time it was accessed, I had to pretend and show J just how nonchalant I felt about all this.

When another surgery was required to remove the port, my reservations were overcome by knowledge of the chemo to come. I never once flinched or hid fear when the Hickman was accessed. I didn't have to. It was painless.

I think of J getting poked to test reaction to the horse serum, and the reminder of what the Hickman was sparing her. I think of midnight on Holy Thursday and the new marrow slowly flowing to where the Hickman sent it; the marrow knew where to go once inside, but it would have been lost without the Hickman. I think of a Boston transplant nurse discovering she could make a kid laugh instead of cry.

Sometime in early fall 2006, as she looked at the counts and the calendar and saw steadily diminishing need, Dr. Whangbo wanted to schedule surgery. I wanted her to explain the hurry. Dr. Whangbo said the Hickman's connection to the world outside J's body made it an infection risk. It had always posed risk, outweighed by circumstance, but the balance was swinging toward trusting J's immune system. This was an indication of success, but I was not up to speed in the transition. Removal of the Hickman required a leap of faith I wasn't ready for. Letting J get on with her life without a tube in her chest ought to have been an inviting prospect, but the Hickman spared her untold violence. That J would be better off without it was hard to accept.

On the morning of surgery, I asked if I could keep the Hickman. No, I was told, and I was, in a way, relieved. It would be creepy to still have it. It'd be one of those things I don't know what to do with but can't quite let go of, like that old crucifix with the secret compartment containing the tools of extreme unction. Better that the Hickman be disposed of in the Operating Room, hopefully by someone with a more sacred touch than that brilliant buffoon with the scalpel in his hand.

In fairness, the surgeon was exceptional in the way we needed him to be. All three surgeons were: Rusty, Healey, and Snape. You'd barely know they did what they did.

As we sat down for a Thanksgiving dinner at Joan's, two days after J's ninth birthday, we celebrated her highest blood counts since we'd started keeping track.

In reporting the numbers, Dr. Whangbo had said, "So much for the aplastic anemia!"

Sarah O'Neill called to invite us to dinner during the Christmas holidays, and we shared encouragement. Her daughter Molly was months into treatment for leukemia. I told Sarah that on New Year's Day we would begin the 10-week process of taking J off of her immune suppressant, cyclosporine. Sarah said such a milestone must feel wonderful. I don't trust milestones, or the feelings they engender, but J was two pounds heavier than the transplant folks in Seattle conservatively hoped she might be come Spring. She was thriving. Knock on renewable resource.

My expectations had long been ablated, but hopes were high. On the last day of class before Christmas vacation, J via robot played Spin the Dreidel with a classmate. J just got "nun." Bupkis, in other words. The kids shared favorite poems. J read Night Before Christmas. She got a standing O. The feedback on Pebbles was awful, and music to my ears.

In early January 2007, I played golf. I hadn't played golf in New England in January before. It was warm enough for shorts.

Within days, I would resume my seasonally affected sourpuss, with the ground frozen as solid as my scowl and my carbon footprint going Sasquatch from SAD lightbox usage. *Lumos!* But it was bright and warm the afternoon J and I celebrated the life of times of a 1994 Nissan Quest.

Were January golf a more frequent occurrence in New England, we might still have that van, but January more typically is a time for road salt, and it was road salt that brought down the Quest. The power steering locked up. Rust opened a hole for the fluid to leak out of, and the mechanic said the hole was just the tip of the salt lick. There was no saving the Quest.

J took the news hard, and I didn't take it much better. She wanted to keep the van and do something creative with it. My mom saved things, and it's not a legacy I treasure, so I arranged for the van to be towed away. I don't get too attached to cars, not since the 65 VW I'd probably still be driving if that kid with his brand-new license hadn't rammed it with his Pontiac when his puppy distracted him like a bygone Blackberry. I got over that, pretty much.

The van was different. A hand-me-down from Jody's dad and stepmom when they upgraded, it served as a sort of utility car for Jody's extended family. The van handled road trips of varying lengths and family configurations. Gerry chauffeured us in it to our Seattle flight. But on many occasions only J and I were along for the ride, for short trips to Home Depot or longer ones to places where Jody already was or would join us, and we had a tradition of making a new music collection annually for our road trips.

They were bizarre collections, bouncing back and forth between J's favorites and mine with the occasional out-of-left-field choice — *The Munchkin Song,* say—thrown in for a laugh. The songs weren't especially Jody's favorites, so when it was the three of us, we seldom played them, opting for something mutually agreeable like classical or Livingston or James Taylor, and if we did play them with Jody, we fast-forwarded through the Pogues' *Fiesta,* which she simply could not tolerate, to Sheryl Crow's *All I Wanna Do.*

The three collections served us well on trips to see J's grandparents in Wareham or the Vineyard and, during the latter, for morning pilgrimages to Menemsha Harbor to visit Crabby. We found Crabby on a beach on the south side of the island and kept him overnight in salt water, and when he seemed not to be faring well, J decided he belonged in Menemsha Harbor, by the jetty, so we made the half-hour drive to deliver him to his new home.

J became attached to Crabby or Menemsha, maybe both, because she wanted to return with some regularity. To repeat the circumstances of our ceremonial parting with the crab, we'd ritually stop by the bakery en route, buy a couple of muffins, coffee for me, OJ for J, pop in a tape, drive to Menemsha and hope for a Crabby sighting. *You've got a real fine love,* John Hiatt would sing. *One I am unworthy of.* Should we fail to spot Crabby, we'd sit on the sand and toss muffin crumbs for him to eat later, because we were pretty sure he was around, just worried about the seagulls making a meal of him, or maybe still mad at us for making him stay in a bucket overnight. We weren't sure.

While in Menemsha, we'd hike out on the L-shape jetty of stacked boulders. J didn't venture far at first, but became emboldened with time. We'd wander down the dock and watch fishing vessels set off or unload, or look for minnows, jellyfish and sea stars in the water. Then I'd say it was time to go and J would ask if we could come back and visit Crabby the next day, and I'd say probably not, and sometimes I'd stick to that and sometimes not. Then we'd climb back in the van and rewind to our current favorite song on our current favorite cassette.

We'd open the sunroof and turn up the volume and drive along listening to U2: *Love, lift me out of these blues. Won't you tell me something true.* To "The Lion King": *And it moves us all. Through despair and hope. Through faith and love.* To Sinead O'Connor: *Went to the doctor and guess what he told me … He said girl you better have fun no matter what you do. But he's a fool.* We'd talk about Sinead and how just about nobody else brings that range of emotion to songs. J sounded better singing along with Sinead than I did.

We decided to donate the van to the public TV station in Boston that sounded like GVHD, though not for that reason. The van would never be driven again, but the usable parts would be of some interest at auction and worth a write-off to us and a grand or two to the station. In the driveway the day before the Quest's last ramble, J climbed into the swing she'd created in the crabapple while I poked around for hidden treasures on the floor, under the seats and in the assorted compartments. J reminded me to save the dashboard ganesh, which possessed parking karma.

We opened the doors and turned up the volume. We listened to Springsteen's *Out in the Street* and sang along to the *oh oh oh oh oh* part. Dan Zanes covered *Polly Wolly Doodle* and the Cowardly Lion sang *I would spare the lash, I would show compash!,* but J had outgrown those and some others and wanted to fast forward. Still, it was good to give the collection a last listen. We decided not to replace the van, to get by with one car and see if that stopped the glaciers from melting. Besides, cassette players aren't standard equipment anymore.

A reporter from the Boston Globe and another from the Brookline Tab were interested in writing about J's experience with Pebbles. We weren't keen on publicity, but the robot was a promising technology that could help kids in challenging circumstances, so we agreed. I told both reporters, and then a brother-in-law, that we seemed to have begun our re-entry. It whiffed of pat response, but by saying it aloud I was coming to believe it. I repeated it because it was true. We were in some transitional return. It wasn't *back to normal,* because normal was a false assumption to begin with, but there was a lowering of my guard, a sense that things were OK or en route to some reasonable facsimile.

The Globe reporter was someone I'd once worked with at the Herald, and so was the Tab reporter's boss. Those sort of small-world connections are common around Boston. When I moved from the massive, more populous and disconnected L.A., those diminished degrees of separation were hard to get used to, but they'd gotten normal over time, especially since watching a stranger's marrow flow through the Hickman.

GVHD was a question of when, not if, and of how severe. Cyclosporine was J's defense, and had done its job well. J had experienced virtually no GVHD, and yet we were glad to begin dosing down.

We were one week into the weaning when J called me into the bathroom and matter-of-factly pointed out three large, dark marks on her thigh. She said she didn't remember doing anything to cause them. The frightful sight jerked me back to that sunny afternoon in our driveway nearly 17 months earlier when Emily told me J was scared and crying and I needed to go to her. Since then, I'd gotten a lot better at masking my reaction. "No big deal," I told J. "Thanks for showing me, honey. Let's check them again before bed."

I was nervous enough already. We had gotten J's guinea pig back the day before, and it felt too soon to me. We had the doctor's OK, and J's joy at having Flower back was obvious, we didn't know what brought on aplastic anemia in the first place, and it seemed wrong-headed to invite a pee and poop machine the size of a Birkenstock back into our home. Jody and J's reading of the doctor saying OK differed from mine. They heard the doctor say it was a great idea. I heard the doctor say, "Well, okay, if it's that important, but be careful."

Jody described me as the conservative parent, which was true, but I was tired of it. So I agreed to Flower's return, set some rules and limits on where the guinea pig could be, and decided that if our home wasn't clean enough, I'd just have to get out the bleach-and-water solution and clean more often.

Now J was in the bathroom showing me unexplained bruises. There were no petechiae that I could see, just the bruises. I told Jody about them when she returned home, and she laughed nervously. That's what she does when a loud and panicked *Oh, fuck!* is somehow inappropriate. It's her Jesus face.

Jody's mother was with us for dinner that night, and as J joined her mother and grandmother for some sewing and a Billy Wilder film, I read the Sunday *New York Times* and thought about what I'd seen. J had ridden that awkward swing we'd hung from the crabapple tree. She's ridden her bike. I preferred those explanations to engraftment trouble or GVHD, and yet aplastic anemia had announced its arrival with bruises from a catastrophic drop in platelets.

I buried myself in a Week in Review story about Congress's new alpha male democrats, and struggled not to cry. I'd been telling family and friends how high her platelet count had been for months, consistently in a normal range. Could they have taken a sudden dive? Why?

I took a few slow, deep breaths, told myself it was the swing or the bike, and read on about some flat-top senator from Montana. The Congress had ex-quarterbacks and cowboys, a first-ever grandma Speaker, but no stay-at-home dads.

Prognosis brightened daily post-transplant, and yet we could assume nothing, As we tapered cyclosporine, rashes emerged, and a topical form of cyclosporine was prescribed. It worked with remarkable effectiveness and speed. We took J's temperature daily for awhile, but came to rely more on perceptions – letting coughing, congestion, lethargy or other symptoms trigger our reach for the thermometer. We wanted our child to feel she was well and getting better, rather than constantly looking for sickness.

When J's illness was at its worst, when the fevers wouldn't abate for weeks, when she was without immune defense and could barely go two days without a transfusion, Jody and I learned to leave nothing to chance. We watched and listened for symptoms of any sort, second-guessed every perception, tried to dose meds right to the minute, right to the cc. I got to be like a neurotic on a windy night sitting bolt upright in bed and saying *What was that?* every time a branch rubbed against the window. The disease and treatment were frightening enough for J without my help.

From early on, J understood the importance of paying attention to what was going on with her body, and that she could take ownership of getting better. There was no one better equipped to handle it than she, and she grasped this. J would suggest we check her temperature, and we would. She tired of me feeling her forehead. She had become so good at reporting anything that seemed amiss, and my obsessive questioning made her nervous. I came to rely on her to tell me what was up with her, and she never failed me.

And so she called me to the bathroom to tell me about the bruises. When it came time for J to brush her teeth and go to bed, I asked Jody to give the bruises a look.

"Are you worried, Dad?" J asked.

"It's like taking your temperature. Just something we've gotta pay attention to. We should take another look in the morning."

I half-expected Jody to see bigger bruises than I'd seen earlier, perhaps even blood, and that we would soon be back in the emergency room. I gave them privacy.

J burst out of the bathroom screaming.

"Hey, Dad, it was ink!"

I don't know where the ink came from. In that way, it was like aplastic anemia. "My pants, I guess," said J. I could hear Jody laughing. Not a nervous, *Oh, fuck!* laugh. Just laughter.

"Mom poked one and asked if it hurt," J said. "I told her it didn't hurt at all!"

A few wipes with a wet cloth and the bruises went away.

J put on her PJ's and came to say good night. She gave me a great hug and said she loved me. *All the way to Fife.* I was incoherent in response.

I like when a wet cloth makes the problem go away.
I can feel J's hug right now.

Pebbles' inventor was eager to visit. Issues of privacy and confidentiality usually prevented his meeting the beneficiaries of his creation, but once we'd been identified in the newspaper, he approached us, and we invited him over.

Michael and his wife, Sarah, were in Boston from their home in Toronto. They came to our home on a Sunday, days before we were to return to Seattle. They took off their shoes and used Purell, and after seeing and hearing what he wanted of his blue robot, Michael entertained us with stories.

There was this one about a "somewhat precious" TV reporter's story about an early Pebbles with a mechanical arm that didn't merely elevate, as ours did, but swung out and up from the side. As the reporter told viewers about a teen Pebbles user, the patient, maneuvering Pebbles' arm via remote control, lifted the reporter's skirt. The reporter kept talking and trying not to seem distracted while brushing at the mechanical arm with her free hand. The cameraman couldn't keep from laughing, or the camera from jiggling. Then the reporter turned and profanely lit into the teen in his hospital bed. The cameraman never stopped shooting, and the tape came to haunt the reporter at a company Christmas party.

On one of J's last days attending school via robot, she told Michael's story. Her classmates cracked up at a volume that overwhelmed Pebbles' audio. Libby cracked up, too. And when calm and two-way communication were restored, she joked that she'd better not wear skirts to class. The kids cracked up again.

Libby realized that J would return to the classroom in a week devoted to MCAS testing. MCAS stands for Massachusetts Comprehensive Assessment System, the means by which the state monitors school performance. We agreed the timing was bad, and that J should return a week later.

J had been out of school for a year and a half, but we needed a doctor's note to miss the MCAS.

The Friday before we left for Seattle, J had her last Pebbles session. Her classmates crowded around the robot; all those smiling, screaming faces, five blocks away and present for the last time in our basement.

"I love those guys," J said, as I reached behind Pebbles and hit the off switch. I looked forward to her return to the classroom. Part of me, anyway. But the next time Libby took attendance, the robot would be gone, J would say "Here!" and I wouldn't hear it, and I'd have to start creating another new normal while learning to trust that my daughter was OK back among the Malfoys.

CHAPTER ELEVEN

Many Happy Returns

W e returned to Seattle a month early. We flew commercial. J faced a battery of vaccines and one more bone marrow aspiration. Jody and I were eager to get her back into school, back into life, which required both the vaccines and confirmation of mature marrow. In a nod to our eagerness and how remarkably well things had gone, Seattle let us return after 11 months. J would return to school just under a full year post-transplant. We couldn't fudge contacting the donor, though; we'd have to wait a full year, to the day.

I promised Jody and J a Lake Union seaplane flight once we'd been cleared for take-off. Indeed, that was part of my Christmas present to them. They still have the hand-written voucher somewhere, but it was never redeemed. We fast discovered it was friends on the ground, not pilots and aerial views, that we wanted.

We stayed with Sarah B. and her family. We saw our original Seattle welcoming committee, Pat and Barbara, for dinner at their home in West Seattle, with its stunning view across Puget Sound to downtown Seattle. We returned to Transplant, said hi to a few nurses, then ate at the Thai restaurant that contributed protein and calories when J's appetite was otherwise on chemo strike. We returned to the Japanese gardens, hiked around Green Lake, and finally saw the aquarium and zoo.

A section of the zoo was enclosed and damp, but the doctors said we could go, so we did. At the aquarium, otters splashed droplets of tank water on us and into the air we breathed. We rolled our eyes and took the blessing.

Doctors wanted only one parent at the vaccine appointment, and J, having ascertained that my feelings would not be hurt, opted for Mom. I wasn't there for her second go-round with her grandfather's vaccines. Tetanus did a number on her. Both thighs ached for 24 hours, and she rode in a wheelchair to dinner with cousin Brent and Jenn and didn't last until the main course. We spent the last few nights in the Residence Inn, mainly for the pool that J had so long been denied. The ban lifted, J jumped right in, and we swam daily. Bender, the science tutor Penny and Sarah B. and her family came to swim and celebrate.

J strapped on a harness and scaled the indoor REI mountain; she went so high, so fearlessly, and impressed Jody and I with her strength and courage.

But the seaplane simply vanished from our list of things to do in between pokes, prods and progress reports. I'm still in the hole for one Christmas present.

We stopped by the SCCA one last time. We didn't have an appointment; we just wanted to say goodbye. A doctor approached us on our way out, in the clinic's rotary driveway, and was pleased to be recognized: Colleen Delaney. How could I forget?

Dr. Delaney was clear, curious, positive, even charismatic, and had a remarkable ability to understand J on a basic and essential level. Dr. Delaney has a mind afire, and she seemed to recognize that quality in my daughter.

A year earlier, at about the time I was packing and shipping boxes to Brookline, Jody, J and I asked Dr. Delaney about what isolation ought to look like back home. Dr. Delaney asked J what she liked to do, and J described our yard, looking for toads and snakes, digging in dirt, taking her guinea pig onto the lawn with her friend Victoria, and exploring the neighbor's pond. I expected, even hoped for, an answer full of empathy and compassion that somehow explained to J that she would do all of that again, but not yet. But that's not what Dr. Delaney told her.

She heard J out, and then she talked to her about the risks for a child with an immune system such as hers—a work in progress, immature, compromised and vulnerable. She told J she wasn't out of the woods but didn't have to stay out of the woods. She talked about ways to dig without throwing dirt into the air, and into her face; about wearing gloves when exploring the pond, and not splashing water. She talked about mold and spores and other things in the soil that cause problems, and why maybe J shouldn't go outdoors on a windy day.

J took it all in. Jody teared up just sitting in on the conversation. I eyed the nurse nervously taking in the boldness of Dr. Delaney's advice.

Jody and I believed in the role of the spirit in J's healing. J.K. Rowling, Roald Dahl and E.B. White provided magical and hilarious places for her to escape to. Tutors engaged her inquisitive mind. Dr. Delaney gave her a way to reclaim her world with eyes wide open, Purell at the ready. She didn't have to be afraid, she just had to be smart. Dr. Delaney trusted her to do that. Here was a doctor who not only cared for J, among the who knows how many kids she treated that day, but took the time and interest to understand her.

I think I would have recognized Dr. Delaney after the better part of a year anyway, but I'd just seen her photograph on the front page of the SCCA's Center News, with a story about stem cells and a successful transplant.

Arriving early at the airport, we found a table in a restaurant and ordered lunch. I got out the newsletter and started to read it to Jody and J. But I lost my composure. I paused, gathered myself, and went on, but again I had to stop. I apologized. I assured J that I wasn't sad, but that the story was too powerful for me to read aloud. I finished it in silence.

It was the story of a 42-year-old Northern California scientist whose acute myelogenous leukemia was growing rapidly and had rendered him suddenly and desperately in need of a transplant. He had no matched sibling, and there was no match in the national donor program, at least in part because of his complicated lineage. In another time, another place, he would die.

Being a scientist, though, and not one to leave this life without a fight, he became aware of stem-cell research in progress at the SCCA. In a lab at the University of Washington, a team of scientists were working with cord blood stem cells. These are not the controversial stem cells, but the ones spilled in childbirth, historically wasted and left to be mopped up, though now more commonly recovered as precious.

Cord blood is forgiving. It is "immunologically naive," so doesn't require such precise matching with transplant recipient, which "increases the donor pool and extends the option of transplant for those patients, especially people of color and those of mixed ethnicity, who cannot find a conventional donor," the Center News reported.

The stem cells captured from one live birth are insufficient for an adult transplant. But the UW scientists were growing cells on a protein known as Delta that could turn a couple hundred thousand cells into several million—enough for an adult transplant.

The Delta stem cells hadn't been tried on a human until the San Francisco man offered himself as a test case. He received his transplant less than two weeks after we left Seattle in July 2006, and it went so well that he'd engrafted and left the hospital in half the number of days as J. Days earlier, there had been no cure. *Time is of the essence.* His desperate need coincided with the opening of Dr. Delaney's clinical trial.

There never is enough time for a Dr. Delaney. The science cannot move fast enough. This is why many doctors opt out of clinical practice, to spend more time in the lab. Dr. Delaney reminds me of Akiko Shimamura in finding a way to do both and make them collaborative. "What draws my interest in science is disease," Dr. Shimamura told me. "There are some very purist scientists, which is great, but that's not enough for me."

Dr. Shimamura once asked for a small amount of J's aplastic blood, not for immediate research, but to hold for when the time came. She admitted it was an odd request, that some colleagues would not approve, but aplastic anemia is a rare enough disease that waiting for the right question before collecting samples would mean slow progress, and we were glad to contribute. If it simply broadens Dr. Shimamura's understanding of a baffling disease, that will be enough.

Dr. Delaney's clinical success was born in the lab of Irwin Bernstein. The emotion I felt in discovering the cord-blood aspect of Dr. Delaney's work, which had nothing to do with our success, was at least in part from my gratitude having our lives touched by such a person. She'd changed our lives, and she was changing the world. She is to Bernstein what J's Grandpa David was to Janeway, and I am in awe.

I couldn't help but to reflect in sadness on the day J and I visited Seven West to say goodbye before leaving for Seattle and the transplant. I had gotten into conversation with a man whose daughter's recurrent cancer demanded a transplant, but there was no match for her—a complication of blood line.

The marrow donor program is the worst bigot I've known. The man's daughter died within 48 hours of J's transplant, and maybe four months before she'd have begun med school. Would expanded cord-blood stem cells have worked? It is a wrenching question to consider. Each year, 16,000 diagnosed with leukemia need transplants but have no donor. Scientists only discovered in the 1990s that leukemia begins in a stem cell. Science will never move fast enough.

J posted: *"Hi people. You're never going to believe this. I KNOW THE NAME OF MY DONOR! I'm glad to say that she seems like a really really really nice person. Anyway, let's get updated. A few days ago, me, my parents, my two Brookline cousins and their mom, Grandma Lucy and Grandpa Gerry, Aunt Linda and Uncle Dave went to Florida for my cousin Susan's wedding! It was so fun, and if you see me in the next week, you'll notice that my nose and face are so sunburned you wouldn't believe it! We stayed at a place called Jupiter Beach Resort & Spa (it's not on a different planet). They have an awesome pool that me and my cousins spent three-quarters of our time in. (In school, I'm studying fractions.) We had a really nice room with a view of the Atlantic Ocean. Today we are back home in Brookline and me and my cousin Emily found that it was toad season in the pond across the street from us. It was so exciting, you should have seen all the toads! Back to my donor. She's 26 and she's from South Carolina. She has curly hair like my mom's, same color too. And apparently she has a really nice family. We got a letter from her mom and she's so nice and sweet that my mom cried when reading the letter. The donor is so nice that she invited us to her graduation when she becomes a doctor. She is going on to become a pediatrician."*

I remembered fludarabine, fluconazole and furosemide, and more or less what they were for, but J didn't need the meds, and I didn't need the names, the amounts, times to be taken or side effects to watch for. What I needed to remember were names of parents of J's classmates. I'd have the rest of the school year to get them right, maybe a whole lifetime. Hard to say.

219

We got a note for the school from Dr. Whangbo, explaining J's absence. That was quite a note.

Jody walked J to school her first day back. I'd join the parade many times, and was glad to let Jody have the honor. And it was a parade, a triumphal homecoming, with a five-block procession to Lincoln School's rotary driveway. Strollers, scooters and bikes shared the sidewalk with pedestrian adults and kids pre-K through 8.

They were just kids again; the Malfoy curse had lifted.

The hallway outside the classroom featured posters and a banner reading *Welcome back J.* Jody and J arrived early, and got in a nice, long hug with Libby before the others arrived. J's desk was adorned with three balloons. She received cards from her classmates. The robot attended, in a newly disconnected state, and J said *Here* without the middleman. She was a little shy, but loved every minute of it.

There was a certain anticlimax to the return. J had been physically attending the school for tutoring sessions after hours twice weekly for months. She'd had occasion to drop by her own classroom and see Libby when the time was right, and once met with her classmates on the playground. And she'd attended via robot.

Resuming everything at once seemed a bad idea. We planned to play it by ear how soon to return to church. That aspect of our world—though it provides J an appreciation and understanding of world religions, why humans are drawn to them, and the value of faith—is more about community than specific theology. When they're thought of at all, Unitarians are the brunt of jokes by the One True Church or *My god is bigger than your god* type. We tend to roll with it, and to consider what it means to be human and whether there's something divine inherent in that.

The congregation and ministers had supported us in myriad ways, and yet I wanted J to wait. But she was eager to return. I thought she might be shy, but she plunged in.

After the service, J disappeared into the crowd with her friend Katherine. Early in J's ordeal, the kids from the Lincoln after-school program made a video of greetings, and on it Katherine sweetly told the story of J being the first to befriend her when her adoptive mom brought her home from the Chinese orphanage. Now they were back together, tearing around, grabbing handfuls of whatever food was available at the public trough, then ducking under the table for their own private party.

The clinging child I'd expected to tug me toward the exit hadn't come with me. Over the next few months, church friends and others marveled at J's confident presence, her willingness to sit at a table full of adults and participate as an equal. She'd sit down at the piano before a full audience of classmates, or a well attended Sunday service, and play without visible nervousness but with a graceful pairing of confidence and humility. Friends asked if her presence, composure and maturity were the result of her medical adventure. I hadn't a clue. She was a remarkable child before, a remarkable child during, and left me shaking my head after. It's shaking still.

Spring is an active time for field trips, and I participated in all available: a tour of Fenway Park, where the Red Sox play and where Jimmy Fund kids have been known to throw the first pitch; a train ride to Boston Common and a historic tour, complete with actors in revolutionary costume and character. I had chaperone responsibilities for J and two others, and as we followed Mrs. John Hancock through the graveyard, I maintained a vigilant watch.

It was wonderful to be back in person with all these former child stars of broadband robot, but by day's end, I was spent. I wasn't in emotional shape for this. Back home, I took a long nap. I was more prepared the next time, for a field trip to the Harvard Museum of Natural History. On the train home, another weary parent said she was looking forward to fourth grade, when parents were less often needed as chaperones. Not me. After missing all of second grade and most of third, I wanted to tag along as often as they'd have me.

J's classmates and room parents threw a wedding shower for Libby in the school cafeteria. Shortly after the school year ended, Libby was married in a Catholic church near the Massachusetts-New Hampshire border. Two of J's classmates carpooled with us, and we drove in a deluge. It rained so hard that an underpass flooded and the low-riding Prius could barely make it through. Ten minutes later, we'd have been stuck. But I pulled to the right shoulder, where the water appeared shallower, got through, and with wiper blades on high we made it to the wedding on time. Other classmates joined us in our pew. The only boy from the class to attend was too shy to sit with us.

Libby was radiant and maintaining her composure rather well as she walked up the aisle, but then she spotted her kiddos, lined up like angels and waving their blessings. As she stood at the altar, surrounded by painted saints and statues of Jesus and icons with haloes, her shoulders shook. Jody and I had tears in our eyes, as well.

In Summer 2007, we went to Southern California to see Aunt WP, my brothers and their families. We showed J where Jody and I were married; it was not the highlight of her trip, placing well behind Disneyland with cousin Sabrina and tide pools with Uncle Dan.

Returning home, J restaked her claim on our Brookline friends' pool and we became reacquainted with Martha's Vineyard, tick checks, and arguments over sunblock. Island neighbor Livingston took J and her four cousins for rides on his motorcycle and sidecar, and taught J to drive his tractor. Once, that would have made me nervous. *I used to care,* Dylan sang, *but things have changed.*

J held front-porch fundraisers and attended a Jimmy Fund picnic with Molly. You've can't be neutropenic at that event, and such was our fortune that neither was lacking in the little guys that day. They cuddled baby farm animals, and instead of reaching for the Purell, I reached for the camera. *Things have changed.* Carpenters began work on J's Make-a-Wish treehouse. I began going through notes and Carepage entries and thinking about writing in the fall.

J got a little tired of hearing how curly her hair had grown in. We traveled to Long Island, where J reconnected with more cousins and Jody delivered a variation on her siblings paper that had taken us to Edinburgh.

Before I knew it, it was Labor Day, two years since I'd learned what idiopathic meant.

I posted: *"Two years ago, back to school time lasted one day. Last year, back to school time coincided roughly with Easter. So next Thursday, when J begins fourth grade, it will be quite a day. Back to school time, indeed. We haven't updated this page in four months; the last time J introduced you to her bone marrow donor. We still haven't met her in person but hope to this fall.*

As for the Carepage, we intend this to be the final posting. J is cured. We're not sure what else to say. I told J this was probably our last posting, and was there anything she wanted to include. She said to make sure to describe the donor ('She's very pretty. She reminds me of my mom a bit, with really curly hair.') She also said I should acknowledge cousins Emily and Michela, who were so important "when I was immune suppressed and I couldn't do anything outside." Needless to say, they're making up for lost time now.

"I took J to the Jimmy Fund Clinic this week because she spiked fevers for several days. It was simply a virus, and her new immune system has since done what it's supposed to do. They checked her blood counts, as always. The platelets have been in a normal range for over a year, and remain so. The red blood cells have been climbing steadily and also remain in a normal range. The surprise was in the infection-fighting white cells, and neutrophils. Both had long been in a safe range, but leveled off well shy of normal. Until Tuesday. Both counts had nearly doubled.

"It was so wonderful to get that report from Jennifer Whangbo, who has been involved in J's care almost from Day 1. Dr. Whangbo had this news, as well: it's time to begin transitioning from the Jimmy Fund back to J's regular pediatrician. We're not eager to give up regular visits with Dr. Whangbo, but nobody said getting back to normal was going to be easy. It sure is welcome, though. Thanks for listening."

Chapter Twelve

Teaching a Dog to Heal

Animal research is the He Who Must Not Be Named of my daughter's cure. Human suffering is a horrible thing to watch, and to watch is to want to do something. *Please, make this go away!* I looked to doctors in desperation and in hope that they could make aplastic anemia go away. And they did. They didn't even understand the disease, not really, not nearly as they will, but they made it go away.

I told Jody who I wanted to write about in telling the story of J's illness and cure, and she suggested it was essentially a list of people I wanted to thank. She was right, to a point. But many of those I want to thank have four legs.

The website of the Chamber of Commerce in Cooperstown, N.Y., cries out to tourists with the Baseball Hall of Fame, Glimmerglass Opera, James Fenimore Cooper. But nowhere is there reference to the kennel to which I trace my daughter's cure.

The Cooperstown Beagle Colony is famous in oncology, hematology and transplant circles, but not so much with the tourists. E. Donnall Thomas performed the first bone marrow transplant in Cooperstown, at the Mary Imogene Bassett Hospital, where he was chief physician. The 1956 transplant gave a twin's marrow to a child with acute leukemia. In preparation, the recipient's leukemic marrow was wiped out by total body irradiation. Progress was slow and agonizing. It was 12 years before a transplant was attempted successfully with marrow from a sibling/non-twin donor. And in 1973, a transplant was successfully performed using an unrelated donor.

In 1979, the Fred Hutchinson Cancer Research Center in Seattle found a match for a 10-year-old with acute leukemia on its laboratory staff—a needle in the haystack. The new marrow engrafted, and Laura

Graves lived two more years before a recurrence of the leukemia killed her. The donor search inspired her parents to advocate for a system of marrow donors, they caught the ear of Florida Congressman Bill Young, and their efforts resulted in the National Marrow Donor Program, which not 20 years later resulted in a staggering blessing of matches for J and one, in particular, considered perfect.

It was considered perfect on a comparative scale of histocompatibility, understanding of which was lacking during early transplants. That tissue typing was understood so well, in matching J with her donor, can be traced to the creation of the Cooperstown Beagle Colony circa 1960, and to the scientific creativity of E. Donnall Thomas.

Weeks after returning to school, J brought a new playmate to class. The teacher split students into two groups. The kids knew to be gentle and not crowd Hutch, our newly adopted dog. There were a lot of hands patting a bashful head and a lot of questions. One classmate asked how old Hutch was. I said she'd just turned three. Another wanted to know why her tail was tucked instead of wagging. She's not used to crowds, I said. Another asked what breed of dog she was, and I said she was mostly beagle but part basset. Another asked about the name, and J explained it was the nickname of the place where she was cured. Hutch didn't like the adventure much.

I took Hutch with me just about everywhere to acclimate her to the sudden movement and noises of our neighborhood.

One morning J and I left Hutch at home and went to Sealey's for pancakes. J said hi to Sophie and found us a booth. Sealey's has its regulars, which in normal times includes us, and another is a gruffly jovial old-timer of the species known as Townie. The Townie had taken note of our dog as we'd been out for walks—tail tucked, startled by noises, surprised by every squirrel, bird, truck, or breeze. "That animal's been abused," the Townie barked.

I was taken aback; so was J. The Townie's a friendly enough guy, and he wasn't trying to be abusive himself, but I didn't care to engage him. I placed our order and went to join J. She was hurt by what she heard. For sure, the dog's tail hadn't yet achieved its upright and wagging position, and she was shy as all get-out. I know the Townie well enough to know he'd spent months getting back to walking more or less upright. He's 70, give or take a dog year, and got a new knee awhile back. That doesn't happen without the surgeon learning how.

Our dog is remarkably quiet for a beagle, but she has quite a tale to tell.

Jody, J and I befriended a hematologist/oncologist who worked in transplant but now specializes in treating and researching a debilitating genetic blood disorder. Away from the clinic, the doctor endeavors to understand the disorder using a hard-to-come-by, specially bred line of mice. Away from the lab and practice, our friend is known to adopt strays of assorted species, which perhaps says something about how the doctor came to adopt us.

The doctor does research involving animals, would rather not, would love a better way and will jump at it when it arrives, as it has for some forms of medical research. But genetic blood disorders need the mice.

The patient outlook is bleak and the payoffs are few and slow in coming. You really have to believe in the importance and potential of what you're doing, and so it helps to be a clinician as well. To see and treat those suffering is a great motivator for alleviating that suffering. The work is painstaking, the pace slow, the breakthroughs and cure off in some vaguely possible future, much like bone marrow transplant in my childhood. The research often seems to go nowhere. Should our friend stop for the sake of the mice, or fear of their champions? Others have. *Please, make it go away!*

The doctor joined us one jubilant afternoon in a public park as we celebrated the apparent success of the transplant, playing tag and reveling in newfound health and friendship. J mentioned that we might get a dog when her doctors said alright. We already had a name: Hutch, for the place where she was cured. I wasn't sure I was ready to take on the daily responsibility of a dog, but the wheels had been set in motion.

"When you're ready, tell me," our friend said, and explained the essential role of dogs in transplant research. The doctor offered to go to bat for us in trying to adopt one. It's not often done, because of the potential for calling unwanted attention to an essential part of medical science that suffers from a fanatic problem. But our friend envisioned us, a transplant family, as a perfect match with a research animal. We like perfect matches.

In late winter 2007, the transplant long deemed successful, I could think of no reason to put off getting a dog – especially this idealized, possibly unattainable dog. Jody and J were all for it. It was a fitting way to celebrate that maybe my daughter had been given back the future we'd once assumed for her.

We asked our friend to see what was possible. Soon I was doing my best to convince veterinarians of what a good home we'd provide, and pleasantly surprised at their wary enthusiasm for placing one of their dogs with a beneficiary of the animal's great gift. There was one dog in particular, with a sweet disposition and a role in transplant research.

We met the vets and the dog in a building necessarily secure and anonymous to protect the vital work done there from the fiercest opponents of biomedical animal research. J had only begun emerging from her long isolation, so it was ironic that before we could meet her new dog, we all had to scrub and don clean gowns and slippers to avoid infecting the dog with some bug from the outside world that might compromise other research animals. But if we had become the ones needing to clean up in the presence of a vulnerable other, clearly our lives were in transition to a more hopeful place.

While the dog warily sniffed around the sterile hallway and coaxed MarroBone treats (*With Real Bone Marrow!*) from J, the vets became comfortable with us. One wiped a tear and admitted he'd never seen one of the dogs with a transplant recipient.

Days later, Jody and I completed forms and received advice, offered teary-eyed thanks to the vet, then loaded our dog in a crate into the back seat next to J, waited for a heavy-metal security gate to open, and drove up a steep cement ramp into the bright light of day.

Hutch took her first walk outside with six inches of snow on the ground. She gave me a look like, *You think I'm going to squat on this stuff?* It was a week or so before her tail came out of hiding and dared to wag. For a while, she startled whenever doors opened suddenly. She was slow to relax around strangers or crowds, but was joining a family emerging from our own bunker; part beagle, part bassett, part metaphor.

She started coming out of her shell with other dogs, and even then she was like a puppy, a three-year-old puppy, awkwardly banging into playmates, testing her voice at the overly aggressive, getting her snout spritzed during an ill-timed, get-acquainted sniff. She became a new dog daily, learning to climb stairs, cautiously warming to strangers, chasing squirrels up trees, and painfully coming to understand the limits of balance on narrow perches.

When I tell our dog's story, some are taken aback, and say, "Oh, she's a rescue!," as if she is another emaciated greyhound plucked from an abysmal existence at the dog track, or scarred pit bull spared more violence. What they don't realize is, I'm the rescue.

There are times J and Hutch are asleep in the window seat when I take a deep breath and stare in wonder at how it is that my daughter came to be so healthy and whole once again. The moment recurs with blessed frequency. I used to watch and tear up. I don't tear up so much now.

I want to do right by this dog; the gratitude I feel is immense. Our neighbor Tracy, a dog whisperer without a TV or book deal but who benefits from no commercial interruptions, noted the steady emergence of our dog's confidence and playfulness as her tail transitioned from comma between her legs to fast-ticking pendulum on a metronome.

Tracy was sympathetic to our dog's history, but then, she's a former nurse and helped raise a diabetic child. The child was treated at the Joslin Diabetes Center, across from the Jimmy Fund, and amid the awesome and vast complex that is Harvard Medicine, where J's late grandfather got to thinking about Haemophilus influeza B and E. Donnall Thomas was an oncology protégé of Sidney Farber.

Diabetes has become remarkably manageable, thanks in part to guinea pigs, not that they get much credit. Neither do mice or dogs get much credit in cancer research. Research relies heavily on generosity, and philanthropic motives have a way of drying up when attention is called to animal research. One woman pursued donating a large amount of money to further the work that had diminished her husband's pain and extended his life. But when she asked if the work might involve animal research, and was told yes, she took her philanthropy elsewhere.

Hutch bonded first with me. I walked her most, took her to the dog park, trained her to do her business outside, helped acclimate her to her new world, and fed her. Mine was the voice she responded to. She curled up beside me when I read, ran to the door when I was leaving, slept next to my side of the bed. She rarely left my side, and was slow warming to others. But over time, Hutch became a family dog.

She surprised me, and thrilled J, the day she left me to respond to J's call. J patted the window-seat cushion, and Hutch jumped up to join her.

Hutch walked to school with us most days and got comfortable with kids approaching her suddenly and in number. She's selective with play-mates, having learned the hard way to be wary of big dogs, but loves to chase and be chased. She runs to the mailman; he carries treats. She still tucks her tail when wary, or when she needs to go, but usually it's up and wagging.

She especially likes to steal another dog's toy; she'll prance off in abso-lute joy, defend her booty, and look at me mournfully when I reclaim the toy for its rightful owner. Her sense of right or wrong is not always clear, which makes two of us.

The gratitude I have for doctors and nurses no longer overlooks the vets and scientists. They're rescue people.

I haven't the skills to discuss this rationally when the other person's feelings are strong. It's like discussing abortion with someone adamantly opposed. There's no gray area, no ambiguity. It's simply wrong, always. I roll my eyes, but I've learned not to open my mouth. They don't hear me, anyway, so I shrug and wimp out. Some of them I love them dearly, but I'd feel closer if they didn't shout down the heretic. They're practicing Catholics. I closed that practice. We have different perspectives on the place of doubt and ambiguity in religious faith.

Early in 2007, in UU World magazine, I read a minister's insightful essay promoting gratitude to religious ethic. UU is short for Unitarian Universalist, something of a religious hybrid and my denomination of choice. Unitarianism doesn't get dogmatic, and I'm not a dogma person. I can even disagree with the minister if I'm so inclined, though I have no issue with the Rev. Galen Guengerich's take on gratitude, morality and ethics. "Morality usually refers to the values we hold and the moral rules we follow," he wrote. "The shadow side of morality is cast by people who create repressive moral rules and try to force everyone else to follow them."

Gratitude, intentionally applied, got me through dark times. When I look at my daughter and her dog, gratitude comes easy. Other times it's harder to access. A two-page animal rights ad, also in UU World, sought my support for UFETA. I googled to find out more, and came upon this: "As people of faith, we cannot stand idly by or look away as, every day, animals by the billions are imprisoned, hunted, trapped, clubbed, harpooned, poisoned, mutilated, shocked, burned, irradiated, subjected to unspeakable pain and torture, and even pushed to the edge of extinction in the name of science, commerce, entertainment or sport – often for no other reason than to satisfy human vanity."

Imprisoned. Poisoned. Irradiated. Pain and torture. Edge of extinction. In the name of science. Human vanity.

The words jolted my system like a bag of methotrexate. I've taken some license here; unlike my daughter and maybe my dog, I've not actually felt methotrexate enter my system.

But with one broad brush, stockyard brutality, overcrowded and over-antibiotic'd coops, dolphins in gill nets and baby seals clubbed for fashion were lumped together with the people who saved my daughter's life, by an organization within my own church.

No wonder those who rely on animals to advance methods of alleviating human suffering are secretive. I'm not even sure writing about it is a good thing. Pardon my Gaelic, but ambiguity sucks.

It is beyond my comprehension how irradiation, forced isolation and chemo drugs that make you vomit, your hair fall out and your mouth become an open sore came to be a formula for hope, rebirth and redemption. But they did. My daughter's alive and well, and our dog gets more credit than I do.

J posted: *"As we speak I'm sprawled out in my dad's loft listening to him type the keyboard as I rub Hutch's belly, and she's falling asleep because she loves it so much. Hutch is cute, sweet, and she still acts like a puppy. And whenever we have roast chicken for dinner like we did tonight, she goes absolutely berserk."*

Hutch's ability to adapt to her new environment speaks to the care she received as a research animal, which compared favorably to the care J received on the transplant ward. Federal law requires this.

But I also attribute Hutch's progress to lessons learned from *The Dog Whisperer*. I know enough to take her regularly to the dog park. Jody and J get on my case when I overreact to an accident. *Hail Cesar*. She's quite the snuggler, and she loves the window seat. It's like it was built for her.

By the time the Make-a-Wish Foundation threw a ribbon-cutting party for the treehouse, Hutch was used to crowds, and she sniffed around the yard amid friends and family. Once afraid of stairs, Hutch ambled up to the second level in search of abandoned morsels.

Molly and J went straight to the treehouse to do homework before guests arrived.

The carpenter attended with his bosses. The architect and designer were there, the latter among the first to try out the climbing rope. Lucy clutched Gerry's arm and said, "This is not a good idea." She seemed to be saying, "Don't test the platelet god." But the designer descended with nothing worse than a red face.

Molly, more than halfway through her two-year leukemia treatment, ate cake and said she hadn't made up her mind about her own Make-a-Wish. Emily was there. Emily must've set a record for most hours on Heme-Onc without getting a poke or a Make-a-Wish. I know two Seven West alumnae who were granted their wish whenever Emily visited.

J raced up and down the treehouse stairs, cut the cake, posed for pictures and thanked those responsible for her magnificent new structure, then dashed off with buddies to investigate life in the pond.

I felt obligated to say something, and noted how much work went into the treehouse, that generosity and compassion erected it in my backyard. I said how surreal it felt to see J receiving this extraordinary gift, and looking like she'd never been sick in the first place; that I loved sharing the day with Molly, whose prognosis was so positive; that thinking of the wish, and eventually deciding on a treehouse, had given J something to look forward to during the darkest days.

You wouldn't believe how many nails are in the thing. The treehouse has had more holes poked in it than ... well, you know. The structure was built to last.

The diabetic kid neighbor put down her cake to check her blood sugar, and our descendant of the Cooperstown 17 pounced and wolfed it down lickety-split. Then Hutch tucked her tail and looked guilty, or at least that's how I read the expression. I probably didn't know what I thought I knew. I'm usually strict with Hutch's diet, more so that with my own. But I wanted to tell her to go ahead and wag her tail and enjoy the cake. She'd earned that piece. As much as anyone on two legs at the party, she'd earned that piece.

CHAPTER THIRTEEN

Under the Big Top

Ten Death Eaters had escaped from Azkaban, and soul-sucking dementors were mysteriously and disturbingly absent. But in *Order of the Phoenix*, Harry Potter had more pressing concerns. He had just blown it big with the lovely and emotional Cho, and on Valentine's Day, no less. He didn't understand what had gone wrong—no wizard, Harry, in matters of love. Alone and killing time, he bumped into his friend, the half-giant Hagrid, who was in a rambling, philosophical mood, unwilling to discuss his fresh head wounds, but he described himself and Harry as a couple of orphans, kindred spirits. *Family,* Hagrid said gloomily. *Whatever yeh say, blood's important.* He linked family and blood so absolutely, as if they're conceptually and essentially inseparable, one and the same. But they're not one and the same. Hagrid's wrong. Blood does not define family. The half-giant needs to rethink this.

I woke up the morning of Passover before Jody and J, let Hutch out to take care of things and picked up the Saturday *New York Times* off the front steps. Things taken care of, Hutch ran inside and did this *Look how many times I can jump really high on two legs* thing she does when food is imminent. I fed her, made coffee, and took it to the sofa to read. It was warm enough to open a window, and a woodpecker probing a dead branch made the morning's only sound.

We'd be driving through Pennsylvania later in the day, and I was reading a story on Barack Obama's last big push prior to the state primary. I wanted him to succeed and end the Democratic bloodletting but didn't get my hopes up. Lucy got her hopes up and put them to work campaigning in Pennsylvania, but we'd not arranged to meet, intending to drive straight through.

When the Bush years began, I would hear about the promise of stem cells but didn't know the embryonic from the hematopoietic, the

God-damned from the morally pure. J didn't need the kind of stem cells the president condemned, thank God.

The Obama story turned from the front page, and as I flipped and scanned pages I recognized a concert photo of Bruce Springsteen, which seemed out of place in the news section. The photo was a few months old. In it, Springsteen performed with accordionist Danny Federici.

I hadn't been at that show, or any Springsteen show for a few years, but the scene was familiar. In my memory Federici is at the organ, spotlighted in silhouette and providing background music to a sermon Bruce is preaching about faith and redemption and rock 'n' roll.

The story accompanying the photograph was Federici's obituary. I knew he'd been diagnosed with cancer months before, and had stopped performing, but I'd read that'd he'd made a recent appearance at a show and it was hoped he'd be back in the E Street Band before long. That's hope for you.

I never did get to the second page of the Obama story. J woke up and came over to snug in on the sofa. She asked what I was reading, and I showed her the Springsteen/Federici photo and told her that on his accordion or Hammond B-3, Federici gave me some good times. I told her his death made me sad, but it didn't hit me hard right away. It hit me maybe a half-hour later, as I fixed J and Jody breakfast while they packed suitcases.

I put on Springsteen's second album, and listened to Federici playing organ on *Fourth of July (Asbury Park)*. I took a few deep breaths. Then I skipped forward to *Wild Billy's Circus,* and this might be the first time a grown man cried to that song. *Oh God save the human cannon ball.* Tears and *Wild Billy's Circus* must be something of a non sequitur. But like so many times over the years, Springsteen's music, with Federici in the background, took me somewhere I needed help finding. *And the ferris wheel turns and turns like it ain't ever gonna stop.* I'd been spacey all week anticipating our drive south. The death of Federici, and hearing *Wild Billy's Circus,* brought the hovering emotion home. We were going to South Carolina. We were going to meet the donor. *Jesus sends some good women to save all you clowns.* It was the first day of Passover, the morning we left.

We delayed starting so J wouldn't miss her first soccer game of the spring. She played great. Back in action, a shutout quarter in goal, focused and playing her position even when action was stuck down at the other end, then up and down the field in search of her elusive first goal. It felt so normal, so frustrating, so us against them.

I'd talked Jody and J into driving. We'd not taken such a drive before, and the long, boring hours of my childhood trips from Southern California to Alberta in the back of the three-in-the-tree Chevy, later the push-button Dodge, when we'd start out in the middle of night to get through the Mohave before the heat of the day, had somehow become treasured memories with the passage of time.

I was the youngest in the car then, and I don't remember using a seatbelt, certainly not that time I was sliding around in the seatless way-back and watched through the rear window as my brother's suitcase soared toward the semi a few car lengths behind us. I didn't know it was Ron's suitcase, but when I stopped laughing I apparently said it looked like a yellow brick, or so the story goes, though we were in Idaho and nowhere near Munchkinland. So I didn't think to tell Ron to pull over and reclaim his wardrobe, and he spent much of the vacation in Calgary wearing the same madras shirt and bermuda shorts. At family reunions, the yellow brick is the story that never dies, but if it ever does, I won't mourn the passing.

One summer we drove to see Nana Peggy for the last time. It was her second go-round with cancer, and surgery had given her a purple face. I need a photograph to remember what she looked like without it. Another time we drove to see Uncle Paul become bishop of Calgary; if Catholicism was more like him, and less like Mom's version, it might still have room for me.

Other times, we drove the 1,600 or so miles just to reconnect with the relatives left behind before I was born. Through the California desert into Nevada, Utah, Idaho, Montana and southern Alberta, there was no FM radio, just staticky AM with nothing on. To bide time, we'd see how many license plates from different states we could spot. Mom would try to get us to sing her Sweet Adeline songs, but she had a snowball's chance in Mohave. Then she'd make us say the rosary, and we'd balk at that, too, but with less success. *Thy will be done.* Prayer still feels punitive sometimes.

We'd see *Watch for Falling Rock* signs in mountain passes, and Dad convinced me there was a Native American named Falling Rock whom I should be watching for. I never did see him. I was pretty naive back then. *Back then.*

I gained a lifelong fear of two-lane mountain roads when Mom two-wheeled it into the oncoming lane around one Montana bend. She must've been going eighty. I was older on that trip. Dad and I drove the rest of the way. It was just the three of us, and the last time we made that drive together.

While Jody, J and I drove to South Carolina, our cat, Carlin Favre, stayed with his favorite neighbor, and Hutch stayed with Tracy, the dog walker who's in my cellphone under Cesar. We'd thought of bringing Hutch along, and the donor knew the story and kind of hoped, but we decided Hutch would be too much of a distraction and probably howl in her crate in the hotel room and get us in trouble.

Tracy also looked after Flower, J's guinea pig, who'd been in a sorry state for weeks, with diminished but still stubborn swelling from a paw infection. She wasn't eating or drinking well, and we'd made a few visits to the exotic animals vet at MSPCA Angell Memorial. She'd lost weight and was still on antibiotics when we left, needing her paw soaked and treated daily. Tracy was glad to help out.

Guinea pigs don't get sick often but are vulnerable when they do. Flower's sister Heart got sick and died in a friend's care early in J's illness. Given that Flower wasn't out of the woods after two weeks of antibiotics, we were prepared for the worst, and warned both J and Tracy that Flower might not survive the week. Uncertain what to do in that event, I punted and told Tracy that should Flower die while we were gone, she should call me and we'd decide then. Flower survived the week, but faced healing of indefinite duration.

J doesn't like it when I refer to Flower as *the pig*. I can call her Flo, for short, or even The Reeker, for the sound she makes when she hears the fridge open or a romaine bag crinkling. *She's not a pig,* J says, and of course, she's right. Guinea pigs aren't actually pigs. They're rodents. And they are a metaphor, though I've also come to use caution with the term as such. I caught J by surprise the first time, and even given her own medical history, or perhaps because of it, she was taken aback by my flip usage.

Guinea pig is a metaphor for research animal. Use of them in this way dates to the 17th century. Mice and rats are the predominant lab animals now, but guinea pigs remain scientifically important in research into juvenile diabetes, tuberculosis and complications in pregnancy. They played a crucial role to Louis Pasteur in the development of germ theory. They were widely used in the U.S. in developing vaccines and antivirals and in the study of immune response to allergic reactions. They played a lesser role in understanding radiation.

Russians and Chinese launched them into space. Czech author Ludvik Vaculik made them an allegory for Soviet totalitarianism. They're on the menu in Peru and Bolivia, and in a church in Cuzco, Peru, a mural by the artist Marcos Zapata has guinea pig served at the Last Supper. Given what Jesus is said to have died for, a powerful metaphor was at work in that art.

When Heart was alive, J and Victoria created a circus for the guinea pigs. When we lived with Gerry and Lucy, J and Victoria would take the guinea pigs into the backyard and let them feast on bamboo. Guinea pigs love bamboo leaves. They also like cover. J would coax me to unbutton my shirt and let them scurry inside to the darkness of my sleeve. She couldn't talk me into it often, but when she did, we howled, for different reasons, but both of us.

But now Heart was dead and Flower was struggling, and as a family we were coming to grips with how far to go with care of a guinea pig. Perhaps an animal whose cousins played such a role in alleviating human suffering deserved all the care available. I'm not sure how to run that equation. But the cost rose with each return to the vet. *Perhaps another set of X-rays?*

We have a guinea pig that never was a "guinea pig," a dog that was, and a cat who's a great mouser adopted from a shelter and named for a comedian and Super Bowl MVP but without any metaphor to call his own. J argued that we couldn't just watch Flower die. She wanted to know how far would we go with Hutch? How far with Carlin Favre? Was there a pecking order among our animals?

Reunion with her guinea pig had helped J through her uncertainty, long isolation and return to health, and their bond was strong. Flower was one of her somethings to look forward to, perhaps the main one.

I proposed, as a solution, that we do right by our existing pets, and agree to a moratorium on additional adoptions. This was a hard choice for J, who loved nothing more than to visit the adoption center at Angell Memorial and see what's available, and regularly conspired with Aunt Wrapping Paper on acquiring her own cockatiel. We never did put a price on how much to spend on any of our animals' health care, but we inched toward a limit.

We handed off the animals and set off for Columbia, South Carolina. We prepared for many hours in the car—roughly 15 there and 15 back, depending on side trips. I didn't know when we'd see the Eastern states from north to south again, and felt the occasion deserved the kind of bonding only a road trip can provide. J brought headphones and bonded with DVDs of *The Bee Movie* and *The Waterhorse* until we unplugged her. Jody brought a collection of stories on CD from *This American Life,* and got to laughing so hard I flashed back to Mom two-wheeling toward oncoming traffic around a mountain bend. Jody assured me she could laugh loudly and drive safely. J read *Nim's Island* aloud, and Jody howled at that, too, but by then I was driving and in control.

Through Connecticut, New York and Pennsylvania, deer carcasses lay off to the side of the road. At one particularly deadly crossing, deer lay on both shoulders. It doesn't take much to make me nervous in a car. I watched the periphery and wondered when a deer would dart out into our path. Priuses aren't made for such interaction. They're better with carbon footprints than hooves.

Deer gave way to crosses. The further south we travelled, the more roadside crosses there were. Tall trios of crosses seemed meant to communicate in code. I'm used to one cross. Maybe the roadside trinity referred to those crucified on either side of Jesus; the merely criminally human, immortalized in *Life of Brian* by Eric Idle's unforgettable whistle. *Always look on the bright side of life.*

We made it more than halfway the first day. We pushed it to optimize time with the donor on Sunday, her day off, and maybe take her to dinner.

We made it all the way to tobacco country, which was a mistake, because only smoking rooms were available at our motel. The residual stench from the previous tenant got J, schooled in the meaning of idiopathic, all worked up. We got an early start the next morning.

We killed time playing Harry Potter trivia. J knew all the answers, and corrected some of my questions. I caught her on the meaning of Lupin's name; I told her lupin was Latin for wolf. She challenged the validity of the question, and suggested it was somehow unfair. She'd been a great sport on the drive, though. Lots of hours, lots of miles. Passing from state to state, she was getting excited about meeting the donor.

Flowering forsythia gave way to flowering dogwood and other colors and blooms. The landscape was extraordinary in Virginia, though heavy rain ruled out a side trip along Skyline Drive in Shenandoah National Park. The pinks and lavenders and whites disappeared in a wall of green in North Carolina. Around then, drivers became territorial and aggressive. A truck pulled by a mobile home had large letters splashed across its back window: *Kick their ass, steal their gas.* We passed warily in the Prius.

I'd had enough of *This American Life* and Jody and J's musical selections. I put on *Blood on the Tracks.* This was tolerable through *Tangled Up in Blue* and a couple of songs beyond, but J complained of a Dylan headache a few bars into *Idiot Wind.* I should have known better, but it was driver's choice, and I was driving. *I can't help it if I'm lucky.* We crossed from North Carolina into South, and I thought about the donor and wondered what to say. *I'm, like, your biggest fan!* There was nothing I could gush out that would communicate my gratitude. As we neared Columbia, J wondered if the donor would give her a hug. I said if she gave the donor a hug, that'd settle the question.

Checking into the Radisson, we wasted no time going to the outdoor pool. Next to meeting the donor, that was tops on J's list. The day was warm enough, but the water was late-April cold. J dove right in. So did I. J wanted to stay in. I apologized, swam to the side and climbed out. My blood couldn't take it.

Jody joined us. We were sitting by the outdoor pool when the donor arrived. Her name: Dr. Kristy Rollins. Jody and J ran and gave her hugs as she emerged through the door. I walked over and introduced myself and went to shake hands, and we did. Then she told me, matter-of-factly, with a bit of a drawl, "We can hug. We hug down here." I have a reputation for hugs in my family, but she wouldn't know that, only having the same blood as one McLean that I know of.

I still didn't know quite what to say. J and Jody went inside for dry clothes, and Dr. Rollins and I small-talked about the area and about her residency. She said she was drawn to working in heme-onc, but it's emotionally draining work with hope sometimes in short supply. She thought she'd join a family practice to work with kids she could watch grow up. Like never before, I could appreciate the choice.

At dinner, Jody and J brought out gifts. We gave her a pearl necklace, a mug and plate hand-painted and signed by J, and a purse from J's piano teacher. Dr. Rollins seemed pleased, a little surprised, expressed gratitude. I'm not sure what we could've wrapped that would've felt sufficient. I asked where her family was from, and she asked if I meant historically or where she grew up. I said I meant historically, and she said she didn't know much beyond her grandparents. It didn't seem to matter to her like it did to me, but I'm a little obsessed in that way; I mean, I can trace my dog to Cooperstown.

If the donor was more concerned with the living than those who came before, I couldn't fault her. Her dad was in one part of the state, her mom in another. She'd had a stepfather most of her life and a great grandparent who was adopted. The lines blur.

J said she and the donor were now related. She called her "family," and said this explained why the donor was so easy to meet and engaging and willing to answer any and all questions.

Some donors want to maintain their anonymity; Dr. Rollins agreed to meet us. Now here was this kid she gave her marrow to who says she's kind of like the sister she never had. The kid's my daughter, the donor is not, but who am I to say? My daughter is my own flesh and her blood, and the future is full of hope. J knows she's connected to something much larger than herself, and that there's something within her that binds her in a unique and profound way to other humans. If she can hold onto that idea, it will take her far in this life, and, then, who knows?

In the graveyard, in *Goblet of Fire,* Harry is locked in duel with Voldemort. Harry's looking for strength somewhere, anywhere, and finds it in the phoenix song: *It was the sound of hope to Harry, the most beautiful and welcome thing he had ever heard ... Don't break the connection.*

Had I been the first-born in my wing of the Clan MacGhille-Eoin, I'd have brought along to Columbia the silver drinking cup that's said to have been handed down to the eldest brother for generations. My first-born dad's break with tradition was to hand women the cup and invite them into the toasts. In-laws, even. He'd surely have handed it to Dr. Rollins, though maybe she doesn't drink scotch. I didn't ask. I'm not sure whether she has a castle, either, though there's a family place near Myrtle Beach.

The next day, we met the donor at the Columbia zoo, where, she told J, there were orange elephants. We looked at her funny, but she spoke the truth. The elephants are orange from rubbing against clay soil.

Her mom sent us a photo of Dr. Rollins as a toddler standing before three tortoises, and twenty-some years later the donor and J stood and looked at the same tortoises. To compare images, you wouldn't think the tortoises had moved five feet in all that time.

We didn't see the donor for the next day and a half. She was on call for thirty hours in the neonatal intensive care unit, from Tuesday morning till early afternoon Wednesday. Two sets of premie twins were born and brought to incubate on her watch. New and precarious lives that needed not her marrow but her hands and heart and mind to somehow cajole and conjure toward thriving.

We met the donor at her townhouse after her marathon shift ended. Her mom and stepdad and sister were there. They'd driven a couple hours for the occasion, and we all went out to dinner at a Southern restaurant. Maybe that's redundant, calling a Columbia restaurant Southern, but this one was Southern enough that J could sample fried green tomatoes and grits done right.

The proprietor, the son of one of the donor's med school professors, came by to chat. We didn't call attention to the occasion, and when he left, we returned to getting acquainted. I'm still not sure what to call the donor's mom, other than The Donor's Mom, or by name. We're not related, except by the blood of our daughters. There's no word for this, other than miraculous.

The donor's mom brought a letter to us from her own parents. The patriarch and matriarch of a family that goes back three generations in Conway, S.C., put it in writing that we're family now. The gathering was celebratory in a low-key way. Dr. Rollins sat at the head of the table, opposite her stepdad, and I directed J to sit beside her. J brought along her Sudoku book and worked on it some as we all talked. We traded family stories and tales of trips to Disney World, where, it was agreed, some rides are scarier than others.

Throughout the meal, we all stole glances at donor and recipient. We were all looking for a sign or something, or maybe just marveling in wonder at this human connection. J never said, *What are you staring at?*, and I'm grateful for that. Nobody brought out Purell, and we ate and drank with a lack of concern that was infectious.

The donor is warm, friendly, but a woman of few words, well chosen, to the point, sometimes drily funny. She's the anti-Aunt Wrapping Paper. She'd whup me at poker, even with the Jesus eyes. She joined the national marrow registry less than a year before she was called into action.

The donation itself was no big deal, she said. It happened on a Thursday, but I knew that; Holy Thursday, it was. She was off work till Monday. Her mom and dad were both with her. As if to prove it wasn't a big deal, she said that after recovery, she'd declined a wheelchair and walked to the elevator. As if to prove her daughter's understatement, her mom added, "It took you twenty minutes to get there!" We laughed.

The day of the harvest, Dr. Rollins didn't know much about the recipient, she said. *Eight years old, 25 kilograms, aplastic anemia.* That was the extent of it. She didn't need to know more to do what she did. I'd call it a selfless act, but what could be more full of self than shared marrow?

There was more to say, though not the means to say it, and we ended the evening fairly early. The donor's family had a long drive home, and Dr. Rollins was about ready to crash from her thirty hours on call. The bill came, and Jody grabbed it. For what we'd received, it was the least we could do.

The next morning we began our drive north, across the Mason-Dixon Line, with a stop at the museum at Jamestown, the original settlement of English immigrants, which J's class had been studying. Near Jamestown, we kept slowing to avoid turtles large and small crossing the road. At sight of the last one, a small one, J convinced me to stop for an inspection.

In the time it took to pull to the side and back up, that turtle had disappeared into the muck, but I saw a head poke out of water, then duck back under, and I called to J to come see. The water was shallow, and the turtle's effort to dig in could not hide the orange spots from our view. The spotted turtle's shell was probably four inches in diameter, and as we studied it, I saw another without spots, about the same size, and we went to inspect that one. J was ecstatic and thanked me for the sightings. But then we had to put them back into the water and apply Purell and resume our drive home, with a planned stop that night at Jody's sister's house—a step-sister, technically—to be followed a day later by another few-hour drive and a visit with another step-sister and her family.

It seems silly to distinguish step-sisters from biological sisters. It clarifies something for the copy editor in me, perhaps, but it also separates in an unnecessary way.

I do think you could take a picture with Jody, her biological sister and the donor, and strangers would have trouble telling which one was not related. The lines blur.

I was asleep in the backseat. Dad was in the passenger seat chewing on his pipe or maybe dozing himself. Mom was at the wheel, driving through the mountains of Montana, and the turn and grade caught her by surprise. She couldn't stay in her lane, and the tires squealed and the force threw us hard to the left and Mom struggled to hold onto the steering wheel and bring it back into her lane, back firmly on four wheels, back to a safe speed. When she regained control, she pulled over, stopped and we changed drivers. I didn't let her drive again on that trip. She'd lost control once and scared the hell out of me. With her foot on the gas and hands on the wheel, my trust was done. She didn't get behind the wheel again, not with me in the car. Faith in a parent is a terrible loss.

Driving along en route to meeting the donor, we listened to a CD of songs from *Charlotte's Web,* so J could rehearse her role as the rambunctious boy Avery in a three-night run soon after our return to Brookline. This was the musical version of the E.B. White farm story of a talking pig, a spider who saves a life with spun words, and the moral consideration of whether it's OK to kill a four-legged runt with dimples to make bacon. I'd like to read Michael Pollan's review of this production.

The cast consisted almost entirely of fourth-grade girls, as boys at this age seem to think singing like this is too wussy, which is what I would have thought at that age but I've changed my position, and now I'm watching three nights in a row and going soft. My eyes are red and weepy, and it's from the oak pollen, no really, and J's up there on stage animated and singing loudly and nailing all of her laugh lines.

The performance group is called PALS, and it's an organization based at J's school but with a roster not exclusive to it. J had been set to begin with PALS in September 2005 when aplastic anemia changed things. The founder and artistic director, something of a local legend, showed up with a T-shirt and a card to let J know she was missed. Over the course of J's treatment and cure and slow return to the infectious world, the artistic director had retired, predictably taking with her some prestige and parental confidence and commitment, and so the PALS J returned to had a gifted and diligent young artistic director but fewer kids involved and a reputation in transition.

Before our trip to meet the donor, I'd heard J complain about the burdensome nature of rehearsals, and I feared that her first year in PALS might also be her last. As much as we wanted her to continue, we wouldn't force it; we'd let her choose. As the performance approached, I was surprised to hear her say that she wanted to try out for Senior PALS. Something had clicked. She could see *Charlotte's Web* coming together, feel the reward of the hard work, and understand the value in the considerable commitment of time and energy.

For three nights running, a home-schooled pixie in pink and pig ears sang an ode to eating that stayed with me for days. My golf buddy's daughter had a starlet's presence and sang so beautifully. J and the den mother's daughter played Avery and Fern like Burns and Allen, and I turned to tree sap in Row 5. The story ended and Wilbur survived, reduced neither to prosciutto nor to heparin. Charlotte died, of natural causes, but left offspring to carry on the friendship with the pig.

My story makes no sense, I suspect it never will, and I don't even know how it ends. My daughter's marrow just up and ceased production. A perfectly matched sibling could have been her savior, but there wasn't one available, so we turned to a complete stranger, a perfect stranger, and got lucky. Sometimes I can accept that, and when I can, the new normal is sort of like the old one, and I'm at peace with this world. Sometimes I can't, and then I look to my daughter for the way forward. She seems to know how to just get on with it, like it's in her blood.

J and her former blood line were alone at the hotel pool when the donor arrived. There were hugs. Then Jody and J went inside to change from their swimsuits. The donor and I sat by the pool and got acquainted. It was awkward. What could I say? This godsend, this myth, had become a young woman of few words basking poolside on a chaise.

"I don't know what to say," I finally uttered. "Thanks."

"No problem," she replied, and smiled easily, and we chatted about pediatrics and heme-onc and watching kids grow up. And then my wife returned with our daughter.

247

EPILOGUE

Fall 2013

A century of science, and more scientists than I'll ever have the chance to thank, are responsible for my daughter's cure.

That said, E. Donnall Thomas is the reason for this book. I don't want to think about the story that might have been, and I don't have to, because of Thomas, his colleagues and their protégés.

I stared often at his portrait but never met Dr. Thomas. And yet he defines for me what it means to be a pioneer. I knew that pioneers shared uncommon vision and the will to overcome obstacles, but I'd not understood in any real way the courage required. Thomas did not go it alone. Along with other scientists and physicians, he had his wife as partner and colleague. But he also had a vision, uniquely his, that in my imagining began in a leukemia ward full of suffering children and hopelessly frightened parents, at around the time I was born, in 1954. And he thought to himself, "I can do something about this." And he did something.

His path was for the stubbornly hopeful but not for the weak. For years, he continued to ask questions and seek answers in spite of vocal opposition from those who thought they knew.

The courage involved is perhaps best understood in a story I was told by the niece of one of his colleagues who had heard her aunt talk about doing research with Thomas, while outside their lab protesters shouted and carried signs with the words "Baby Killers!" I'm pretty sure the ones with the signs never went from room to room in a leukemia ward circa 1954.

There was no cure for my daughter's illness before Thomas and his colleagues found one. There's an ever better cure now. That the cure improves, almost by the day, is part of his legacy.

In noting his dying, in Fall 2012, I am grateful that he lived.

I passed Dr. Michael Shannon on the sidewalk on his way home from Boston Children's Hospital, just a long block from where Dr. Thomas had apprenticed under Sidney Farber. Dr. Shannon had long served as chief of the Emergency Department, but as we spoke in early 2009 he was creating a department of pharmacology, taking science to another level to better tailor drugs to the unique needs of individual children. I was on my way to a meeting of the Community Voices in Medical Ethics. He was intrigued, but we hadn't time to complete the conversation, and we never did.

The last time I saw him, he was choreographing my daughter and other children in a performance of Benjamin Britten's "Noye's Fludde" inside a church. Getting children safely on board is how I remember Michael. That he is missed so terribly, by so many, is testament to his capacity for care.

Dr. Kristy Rollins practices pediatrics in Columbia, South Carolina, in her own ways carrying on the legacies of Drs. Thomas and Shannon. She's a gifted quilter. We're Facebook friends.

The Seattle approach of reduced radiation in conditioning patients for bone marrow transplant, for aplastic anemia and certain other hematologic diseases, has been widely adopted at American transplant centers, including the Dana-Farber and Boston Children's Hospital.

The term safe assumption is largely gone from my vocabulary, except maybe when I'm tired or otherwise not thinking clearly. And the word cure is brutally hard to trust. And yet aplastic anemia is a distant memory for my daughter.

She is in high school, studies piano and voice, composition and music theory, explains physics and calculus to me with patience and faith that maybe someday I'll understand. And she sings a mean version of "Angel From Montgomery," accompanying herself on ukelele. "Just give me one thing," she sings, "I can hold onto."

Her physical growth comes in spurts but is considered normal for her age. The radiation avoided seems to have allowed for this normal growth, and for normal development and function of the essential parts that add up to being human.

Her follow-up visits to the Jimmy Fund Clinic have been reduced over time from monthly to semiannual to yearly, and we might even cut back on that. The platelets and red cells and white cells we monitored so obsessively have been in a normal range for several years. Graft-versus-host disease is something we watch for but never see.

We continue to test something called "chimerism." The way I understand it, chimerism is an accounting of her blood: how much is my daughter's and how much is her donor's. The share that is my daughter's is negligible; her blood line, at least with regard to actual blood, belongs to her donor. This is a good thing. Vital, you might say.

The only problem with fewer follow-up visits to the Jimmy Fund is seeing less of Dr. Jennifer Whangbo. I'll miss seeing her, and remembering that afternoon spent looking for neutrophils through watery eyes in the microscope in her lab. I'll miss watching her own children grow up through the photos that she shares.

I guess those follow-ups are not so much about my daughter anymore. They're about me.

About the Author

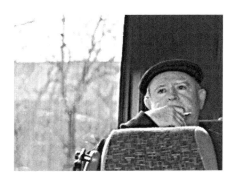

Paul McLean was a sports writer at the L.A. Daily News, an editor at the Hollywood Reporter and Variety, and arts editor at the Boston Herald before finding his most rewarding role as a work-at-home dad. Since 2008 he has worked with the Boston nonprofit Community Voices in Medical Ethics and its affiliate Community Ethics Committee, helping the teaching hospitals of Harvard Medical School better understand and appreciate the people and values of the communities they serve.

He blogs at www.medicalethicsandme.org and paulcmclean.com, and is author of the forthcoming *BEST INTERESTS: Stories from the intersection of life, choice and medicine.* He lives with his wife and daughter in Brookline, Massachusetts.

Made in the USA
Lexington, KY
07 January 2014